HAVE NO FEAR, THE LION SLEEPS TONIGHT

ALTERNATIVE OPTIONS FROM THE LONGEST SURVIVOR OF BONE CANCER

DEBORAH BENEFIELD

CONNIE MACKENZIE

Connie's story—her battle with cancer which shares a twenty-five year journey into Alternative Health Care in the United States.

By Connie MacKenzie

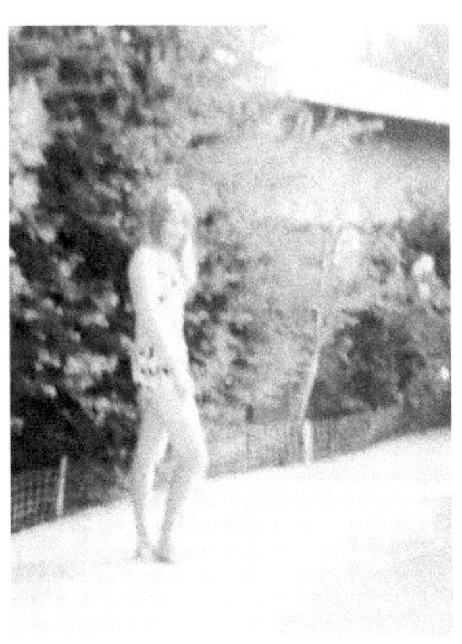

ACKNOWLEDGMENTS

To my mom, thank you for giving me life. Showing me what true strength looks like when you're fighting for your life. You are the strongest person I have ever known. I know you fought for my brother, myself, and my dad. You fought so we would grow up with a mom. You always wanted kids, and I'm so happy you got to see my brother and I grow up. I have so much appreciation for you as an adult. I wish that we could have had a closer relationship when I was growing up. I have you in my heart forever and anytime I want to feel close to you. I listened to your favorite songs, by Olivia Newton John, the entire time I was working on our book. Her singing made me feel you were right next to me, writing with me. I am happy to say; I am more like you than I thought. With much love, your daughter Deborah.

To my brother Benjamin MacKenzie, you were 3 years old when mom got bone cancer. Growing up, the only world you knew included taking care of mom. I just want to let you know how much I love you and I thank you so much for being there all these years for her. Back then, I stayed away as much as I could, leaving you with all the responsibilities of helping her. You had to do things that grownups will never have to do. You never complained, you always made her feel so loved and cared for. All the operations, Doctor's appointments, breakdowns, all the sacrifices you made for her make you one of the most special brothers and sons a mom could ask for. I am so happy you and your beautiful wife Kristy were with her at the end of her transition in life. With much love and appreciation, your sister.

To my Dad Bruce MacKenzie, dad I remember the 1st time I saw you cry after you were told mom had 6 months to live. I will never forget that moment, I really didn't understand, that was the worst day of my childhood everything changed after that. I can say that most men wouldn't ever be able to do all that you did. You worked, took care of mom and tried to raise a family the best you could. I love that you were very supportive of helping mom with all her businesses and dreams. You did her hair make-up, held her when she needed to cry, you cried with her, made her laugh and tried to make life as easy as you could for her. She loved you so much and was so thankful she had you for 46 years of marriage. We will get that medical invention out on the market at some point. Love you dad, I will always be daddy's little girl!

Thank you to all the friends that helped my mom and family on this journey. I know some of you really struggled that I wasn't the daughter that everyone thought I should be because you told me so. I appreciate all the adopted moms and dads that saw how much I was struggling and hiding all my pain and took an interest in me and tried to help me have a happy childhood. You made a big difference in my life. Thank you for all the friends that made life fun and a joy to be around when I was holding all the pain in and didn't share. Somehow you just knew and didn't make me have to think about anything but fun and having a childhood.

Thank you so much to the team that helped me get this book out in 3 weeks so we could meet a deadline and all the encouragement you gave me or just the motivation. Very special thanks to Tara Farquhar Author and friend for 10 years, Eric Lofholm, Jill Lublin, Randy Peyser, Ashley Preciado, Ash Balakrishnan, Joygrace Harmony, David Ament, Tiffany Shockley, Joe Ross, Nancy Lopez, Becky James, Joseph Lazukin, Sharon Hawkins, Sunshine Allred, Oginga Wilson, Lori Smiskol, Tammie Sokoloff, Marcia Wakefield, Tommy Watts, Debbie Ross, Jason Webb, Uncle Jeff MacKenzie, Aunt Shannon MacKenzie, Desiree MacKenzie, Alysha Pitcher, Natalie Raub, True MacKenzie, Randy MacKenzie, Maria Speth, Veronica Rozenfeld, Aaron Young, and all my networking organizations including Berny Dohrmann and September Dohrmann Founders of CEO Space, Ryan Long and Michelle Marie Matich Founders of City Summit, and Greg Reid Founder of Secret Knock that are always there to help.

FOREWORD

While attending a conference in Tampa, Deborah got a call from her family in Houston telling her she needed to get home right away if she wanted to see her Mom before she died; she didn't have long to live. Deborah sat in shock, recalling the last time she heard those words. She was only ten years old! Deborah had been waiting for the day those words would finally come true.

Processing this sudden news, she decided to go to Houston the next day, hoping to get a good night's sleep. She needed to be strong for her mom and the rest of the family. She left the conference. Walking outside, she tearfully reflected on the last thirty-three years, remembering all that her Mom survived in her fight with bone cancer.

Deborah tried many times to move on with her life and put these memories behind her. A few years back, she started to write a book about being raised by a parent with cancer, the effects it has on the family, and the decisions the children make that impact them into adulthood. Deborah wrote her thoughts and feelings on this topic, which gave her clarity. However, she had no idea what was about to be discovered. Years after Deborah had stopped writing, her Dad called to tell her he found the book her Mom wrote years ago. She was totally shocked as she was unaware that her Mom had written a book. A book Connie (Deborah's mom) had written about her 25 years of battling bone cancer and the alternative route to wellness she took.

Deborah was excited and decided to combine her book and her mother's. She immediately started writing again. This time she uncovered even more clarity. In particular, she realized why she and her Mom struggled to have a good relationship. During that time, Deborah was struggling to maintain her 20-year marriage. Being in such a stressful situation, it became too much for her to handle, so she again stopped writing. She never gave up on her goal to complete their book. So, here it is; their combined story, published in honor of Connie MacKenzie.

ABOUT THE AUTHOR

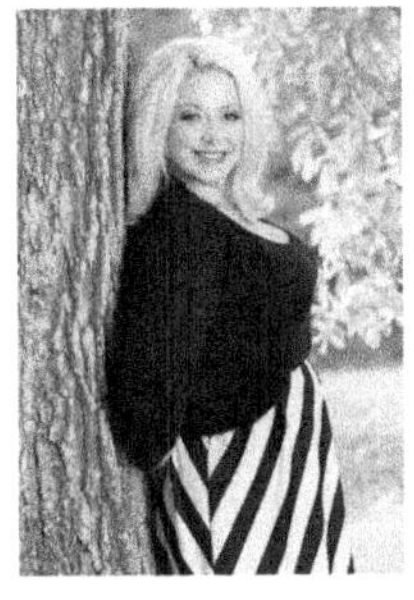

At ten they diagnosed Deborah Benefield's mother with bone cancer and given six months to live. That moment changed Deborah's life forever. Deborah took on the responsibility of her Mom's disease, thinking she caused it. Unfortunately, this belief made Deborah's relationship with her Mom challenging. She shut down and focused on everything except her situation. Years after becoming an adult, she wrote about the efforts of growing up with a parent who had cancer, and considered writing a book. About three years later, her father found the book her mother wrote. This story is mainly Connie's story and covers over twenty-five years of her battle. However, family members also face many challenges and I included some I faced in this book.

Websites:
    havenofearthelionsleepstonight.com
    deborahbenefield.com

ABOUT THE AUTHOR

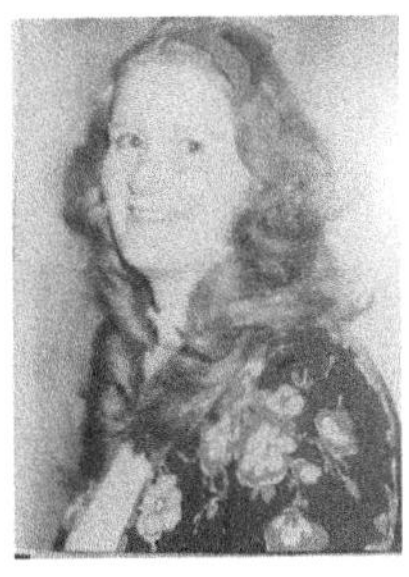 Connie MacKenzie has indeed partici-pated in her fight to recover, as this story shows. Connie had no name, no fame, no riches - only a story of success. She fought a battle for over 30 years against a common enemy, cancer. Orthodox medicine offered her only one hope, a mutilating surgery that would have left her an invalid for life. Using many branches of alternative health care, her own body helped fight the cancer. Many of these various methods are being used by qualified health care professionals today. All can benefit by following her story. By using the methods she did, they may spare themselves from ever developing the disease.

CONNIE'S CHOICE

She is fighting a battle against the common enemy cancer, but with an extremely large and unusual type of tumor. Orthodox medicine offered her only one hope, a mutilating surgery which would have left her an invalid for life. She made an unconventional choice. Using many branches of alternative health care, her own body is being helped to fight the disease. Qualified health care professionals have successfully used these various methods. With one out of three Americans likely to get cancer. All can benefit by following her story, as she is hoping to spare many of ever developing this disease. Connie hopes people consider these alternative choices in treatment before decisions need to be made.

Decision time for Connie came early and shaped her life. In high school Connie became interested in health. Being a native Californian, it exposed her to many preventive health ideas. Connie lived with a slight limp for several years. At twenty, she went to several doctors to find out-Why the limp? Why? A common question which led to an all too familiar trial.

They suspected as a child she had undiagnosed polio as a child or possible Multiple Sclerosis. They made no definite diagnosis. In three separate car accidents, Connie received whiplash three different times. She learned about living in pain during those years. With Chiropractic care, she recovered. With the third whiplash, Connie went to a chiropractor who specialized in soft tissue techniques. He incorporated acupressure into her treatments. The treatments helped her back pain, but the mysterious limp was still there.

In Connie's case, her leg was x-rayed at birth. They feared she had broken during her breach birth. A fall at fourteen while ice skating made her leg even more prone to a tumor forming there. Breach births, falls, and whiplashes; familiar words to many of us. Connie limped down the aisle at her wedding. She took care of herself, yet they discovered no diagnosis.

In 1976 she removed herself and family from all artificial flavorings and colorings, and most preservatives. Her daughter's pediatrician diagnosed her as being hyperactive, and her daughter's allergy tests found her sensitive to these things. With these substances removed from her diet, her daugther's hyperactivity was controlled. Little did Connie realize how a preventive diet for her daughter's hyperactivity helped her control the growth of the tumor in her body. Connie also followed the Weight Watcher's diet for over five years. She had been a lecturer for Weight Watcher's for over three years at that time. This diet is similar to the anti-cancer diet recommended by the American Cancer Society: lots of fresh fruits, vegetables, low fats and no sugar, additives, or preservatives.

In June 1986 her leg blew up like a balloon. An X-ray revealed a very large bone tumor. Fear fell over her when she saw the x-rays. For years, family and friends thought Connie had been pretending to be in pain to get special attention. Familiar, identifiable words. Now with the X-rays it seemed strange, but she had a sense of relief. Finally, proof that she had been in pain all those years, and had not been pretending.

Decision time came in November 1986 at one of the country's largest cancer institutes. They confirmed her fears, but she had not anticipated what she was about to hear. They called a special meeting of many of the department heads. The doctors agreed they had never seen, even in a textbook, a bone tumor of this size. They assume it took over fourteen years to grow the twelve inch by three inch by five inch tumor that rested in her right femur and extended into the hip area.

At the decision time, a hemi pelivic 'dectomy was the only suggested treatment. That meant surgically removing one half of her hip and the entire leg. She would become an invalid if she lived through the surgery and the treatments that followed. Familiar, identifiable words to many people. Connie MacKenzie stood on her feet and walked out of the tumor clinic feeling triumphant. She said "no" to surgery. But a fear fell over her. She asked herself, What do I do now? Walking on her own two feet, she conquered her fear and began intensive study into alternative avenues of health care.

They asked her to return to the tumor clinic for regular follow-up visits. They wanted to follow Connie's case, her impossible case. Every six months she continued to return. Each time she experienced a sickening feeling of fear at what they could find. The doctors say that this type of bone tumor usually spreads rapidly to the lungs. Unfortunately, when one is diagnosed as having cancer, most friends and family call and say goodbye at a time when they are needed most. So, one fights on alone. Life becomes precious since it might soon be lost. Connie was determined to live as long as she was alive.

For a year, as she lay in bed, her mind walked through countless pages of avenues on health. Stimulate the immune system, help the body fight its own disease. Stress produces Pain. Connie's choices came into play. We have found there is a cancer personality profile. Unsolved stress is almost always present at least six months to two years before the illness system, allowing cancer to take root in the weaker areas of the body. For reducing the Stress-Pain conflict, Connie's clinical psychologist found a new and rewarding approach. Using precision muscle testing, he helped her identify her own genuine feelings to emotional stress. Some experts believed that every physical problem has its roots in an emotional cause. Blocked emotions equal blocked energy within the body. Blocked energy surfaces in leading to pain. He helped to identify and correct her energy blockages. "Clearing out," the direct route to unclutter the mind chatter.

The results impressed Connie. She preceded to study these techniques for the following year and a half. She became a certified instructor in some of these great stress control techniques. Before facing the suspected, dreaded decision time, this knowledge provides an alternative life-style. Prevention can avoid so many heartaches.

Connie's husband, Bruce, shared these thoughts with me:

"We cried, we had to let her go. We cried again, but Connie's determination to live drove us to teamwork. Through the trying first year, so many things to relearn."

Father for Bruce, their eleven-year-old daughter Debbie

and five-year-old son, Ben faced new roles. They had to learn to live with the fact that their mother might not be with them as they grew.

Connie took courses to help her learn how to deal with the stress of her illness and to help control her pain. She graduated from The Accu-pressure Connection School in California, a state-approved courses for nurses. She then graduated from the State Certified Houston Massage Center, where Maxine Petteway was Director. She became a state-registered massage therapist. All her instructors were great in working around her physical handicap. She was still on crutches at this time. One of the more difficult times at school was working from a wheelchair during the dissection laboratory class. Connie's way of dealing with pain was to live a useful and productive life even though the State of Texas considered her permanently disabled. Helping others in pain became an important part of her therapy. While helping others she helped herself in so many ways.

They teach massage therapists to help those in pain or under stress by touching and working tight sore muscles, using many techniques. Connie is qualified in this area.

With Connie's diagnosis, it was impossible that she was still alive. This 'impossible possibility' went on with her life. Finishing multiple schools and getting proper state registration became Connie's Goal. She wanted to be qualified to share what she had learned.

Connie, a woman determined to take what she has learned from a trying situation and incorporate it into a medical setting. Her company was Medical Rehabilitation Clinic located in the Doctor's Pain and Stress Clinic.

Connie's choice, a challenge. Her tumor is still one of the largest known in medical history. But something was happening, Connie's story continued. Connie MacKenzie participated in her fight to recover, as this story clearly shows. She had no name, no fame, no riches, only a story of success. Connie's choice not to be an invalid needs to be heard. A friend wrote to Gilda, hoping she would include Connie's story in her forthcoming book. The note below was received from Gilda Radner. It was too late for Gilda. It is not too late for others.

A Note from Gilda,

A hope, Dee your letter arrived. Continue to participate in your fight for recovery. You are not alone.

Much love,

Gilda

INTRODUCTION

Have no fear, the lion, cancer, sleeps tonight!

Our bodies, like a vast jungle with rivers and channels flowing through our veins. We are truly, marvelously made with our built-in hunters continually on guard watching for any invaders that could harm us. We have built-in scavengers that quickly dispose of any slain intruders. Each day our immune system destroys mutated cells that could become cancer if not quickly overthrown. As the cells mutate at an increasing level, they sometimes overcome our hunters and cancer takes hold like a vicious lion refusing to let go.

When the fearful lion attacks, one embarks on a journey, one that often leads down many roads. The unwilling traveler will not return from this journey without great reflection on the future course he/she will travel.

This is the story of a young wife and mother who at thirty-three years of age heard the lion's roar in the distance and then felt its vicious attack while it tried to tear her apart.

She would not be overcome! Yes, don't be afraid because the lion does sleep tonight.

It is my sincere desire that this story inspires others to keep the lion at bay and hopefully to put the lion to sleep long before any diagnosis of cancer.

1

THE LONGEST JOURNEY

I received my diagnosis of bone cancer (Osterosarcoma) in December 1986 at The University of Texas M.D. Anderson Hospital in Houston, Texas, one of the leading cancer hospitals in the world. Five years later my right leg and hip were removed along with half of my pelvis. They formally call this amputation a radical-right hemi-pelvectomy. It has been ten years since my diagnosis and five years since my surgery. Yes, the cancer caused the loss of my limb, but only after many years of the hunters in my immune system holding the lion at bay.

Fortunately for me, a fine man and surgeon, Marvin Romsdahl, M.D., PhD, F.A.C.S. became a very experienced hunter of the lion. He and his assistant hunters helped rid my body of the vicious beast once and for all during a thirteen hour surgery without the use of blood. I am now cancer free and can walk with an artificial prosthesis and my three wheeled walker.

Come, let me take you back in time with me. Together we will share in an unforgettable journey—one that will hopefully help put the lion to sleep forever.

I was born in a breech position on June 20, 1952, in Eureka, California. They feared I broke my leg and took an x-ray. This early exposure to radiation undoubtedly contributed to the osteosarcoma. Remember, x-rays in 1952 emitted much more radiation than x-rays do today.

At age fourteen I fell while ice skating and they took me to the emergency room, my knee and leg in significant pain. My knee was x-rayed, and they found no break. They suspect this trauma to my leg contributed to the outcome of osteosarcoma. When diagnosed, they told me this type of bone cancer is usually found in teenagers. I had symptoms for many years before the final diagnosis. How long had the lion been sleeping?

I became interested in health and nutrition at an early age. My mother had been a nurse and was very interested in preventative health ideas. A national health care revolution began in the sixties and since I lived in Pleasanton, California, the San Francisco Bay Area which exposed me to the pioneers of the new health movement. Adelle Davis, one of those pioneers, wrote several books heralding the benefits of nutritional supplements. Her books were only out-sold by the Bible for several years.

Dr. Shaklee, in the Oakland Bay Area, formed the first company marketing nutritional supplements and cleaning products that were not harmful to our environment. He used a multi-level marketing system. Dr. Shaklee taught people the nutrients their bodies needed to maintain good health.

At seventeen, I became one of his youngest distributors. I was not a financially successful distributor, but it exposed me to a tremendous amount of educational information on nutrition. I remember hearing personal experiences of those who benefited from proper diet and supplementation.

Linus Pauling began sharing the benefits of vitamin C and early in his career but received criticism from the medical establishment. Many years later they praised him for his findings and they consider him one of the brave pioneers who helped blaze the trails of the so-called health care revolution. Today we understand that vitamin C is a powerful antioxidant and free radical scavenger. The vitamin improves our immunity against viruses and helps to stop the formation of carcinogens in our bodies.

Today, there are many advertisements in magazines telling us of the benefits of antioxidants A, B, C, D, E, selenium and zinc. In those early days of the health revolution, they thought the idea that our diet or supplements could help our bodies fight off the lion was ridiculous. Now there is so much scientific evidence that they accept these ideas as fact. In 1997 The American Cancer society awarded Dr. Waun Ki Hong of M. D. Anderson Hospital, a Clinical Research Professorship. He is an international leader in the emerging field of chemo-prevention. His group has shown that synthetic forms of vitamin A, known as retinoids, can reverse the precancerous condition of oral leukoplakia and can help prevent the development of new cancers.

Some in the natural health field have shared reports of people with cancer improving after massive doses of carrot juice, of which vitamin A is one of the main nutrients. As new scientific evidence increased, what they once considered part of the radical health movement has now entered mainstream America. For example, Vitamin E became a popular supplement during the sixties and early seventies. Today they know vitamin E to be one of the main antioxidants that fights free radicals, a process that helps our bodies fight off the lion and many other uninvited intruders.

I always had to watch my weight and tried several diet

programs in the early 70s. With one, I remember boiling down tomato juice to make my tomato sauce and substituting bean sprouts for pasta. As they say, "You've come a long way, Baby", and that statement applies to many of our weight programs today.

As the science of nutrition has grown, we have learned much about the benefits of the different food groups.

It was not uncommon in California in the sixties and seventies to hear of someone having their eyes read to determine the overall health of their body. Frankly, at the time it sounded a little hokey to me. Bernard Jenson, D. C., N. D. of California was and still is a chief proponent of the Science of Iridology (iris analysis). He is almost ninety today and encourages the use of computerized cameras to help note areas in the iris that show signs of chronic or degenerative problem areas. This practice is used by the equivalent of our naturopathic doctors in the European countries.

The problem with alternative health care is that some practitioners are involved with invalid scientific practices and properly recognized training schools have been almost nonexistent. This is changing—twelve states in the United States have already licensed naturopathic doctors and they now recognize them for insurance reimbursement in the state of Washington. Our nation is becoming more prevention minded as practices such as acupuncture and massage are being recognized as valid medical sciences. We will explore several types of alternative health care practices while on our journey.

THAT MYSTERIOUS LIMP

I graduated from Amador Valley High School in Pleasanton, California, in 1970. While attended business college in Hayward, California my Prince Charming swept me off my feet. We married May 15, 1971. It was obvious I had a slight limp in our wedding movies. My friends remember that I developed that limp a couple of years after my high school ice skating accident.

My husband, Bruce, and I were living in Texas in 1972. I had no pain, yet I wanted to know why I had that mysterious limp. The family doctor referred me to an orthopedic who believed I had undiagnosed polio as a child. He ran more tests. The tests showed possible multiple sclerosis, and he referred me to a neurologist. He decided I had one leg longer than the other and might need back surgery. He wanted to wait six months to see if the condition worsened.

Since we married two and one-half years before, Bruce worked as a paint store manager. His work transferred him to California, and I went to a Chiropractor in Sacramento, California. Many still considered chiropractors 'far out' in the early 70s. He agreed with my earlier diagnosis, that one leg was longer than the other, and prescribed a lift to fit in my shoe. He told me not to walk without it. After x-rays, I received a series of treatments over several months and my lift went from three-fourths to one-fourth inch. He released me, told to wear the shoe lift, and to come back if I needed an adjustment. Relieved, we believed the problem was behind us.

Was the mysterious limp an early sign of the lion's presence? As we continue, it will become apparent why it took so long to discover the lion's presence.

In the fall of 1973 I became pregnant. We were overjoyed. Then, at two and one-half months pregnant, in a traffic jam, a car rear-ended me going at least forty-five miles per hour. As often occurs with whiplash, there was no immediate pain after the accident. Regardless, my husband took me to the chiropractor within two hours of the accident. Taking precautions to protect the baby from radiation exposure, he took an x-ray and gave me an adjustment. The next day I hurt all over. They transferred my husband to Kent, Washington during my regular treatments. In Washington, I continued my treatment plan with a chiropractor who was also a naturopathic doctor.

As my baby grew within me I experienced tremendous pain across my lower back and hip area. The pain radiated down the right leg. Fortunately, the chiropractic treatment helped control the pain, and I didn't need to take pain pills that could affect the baby. Naturally, I read and followed Adelle Davis book *Let's Have Healthy Children*. I studied books on childbirth and practiced the Lamaze childbirth relaxation techniques. My mother and sister had been in labor just a few hours before their children were born, therefore I was optimistic childbirth would be easy.

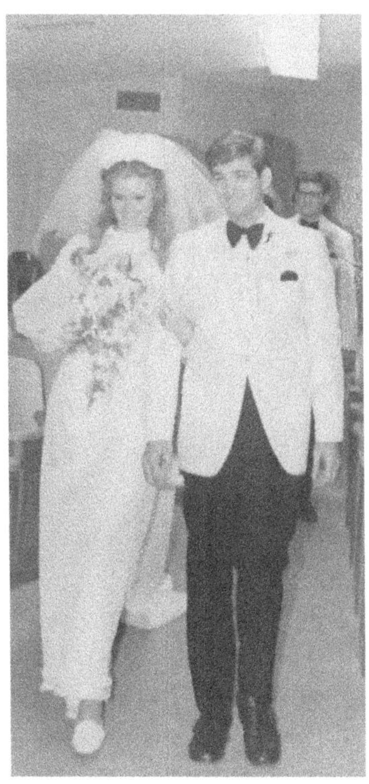

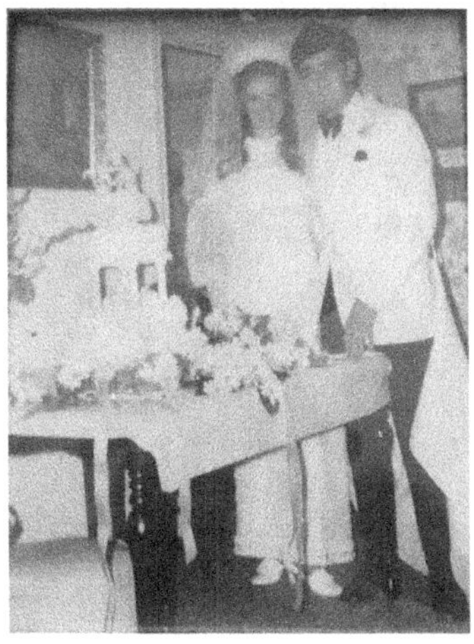

OLD HOME WEEK

When I was seven and one-half months pregnant, we moved back to Pleasanton, California. Many of my friends and classmates were pregnant, too. Lamaze classes were just becoming popular and if the husband attended with his wife, they allowed him in the delivery room. Past generations of fathers were happy to pass on that experience.

The La Leche League, a group furnishing information on nursing, was especially active in California in the 70s. At that time, they considered nursing your baby a backwards movement, and not for the modern liberated woman. Thanks to support groups like the La Leche League, the nation realized the benefits of nursing. Now, they encourage all new mothers to nurse their babies, even if only for a brief time. The rich colostrums given off by the mother before her milk comes in is full of antibodies that help strengthen the newborn's natural immunity to many diseases. It is one of the best things we can do to keep the lion sleeping. Also, a special bonding occurs between the mother and the newborn being breast-fed. Some suggest that mothers who breast-feed decrease their own odds of developing breast cancer.

One month before delivering my daughter, I developed toxemia. I was in a recliner with my feet up for two hours and then I was up for one hour. My OB-GYN told me to take vitamin B6 for fluid retention and avoid eating any salty or high sodium foods. He said he would admit me to the hospital if my blood pressure didn't go down in forty-eight hours. I had lost ten pounds of fluid when I went back. I still rested with my feet above my heart, but I was fine for delivery.

Since I experienced false labor for more than a week, I wasn't sure my labor was real when my contractions started. I took several tablespoons of liquid calcium and magnesium and on to the hospital we went. My water broke on the way to the hospital and when we arrived, they discovered my baby was in the breech position. They rushed me to x-ray and then to the delivery room. My eight and one-half pound daughter was born vaginally in a left footling breech position ten minutes later with no time for the anesthesiologist to arrive. I only received one shot of novocaine for the episiotomy. I contribute the ease of delivery and my relative calmness in a large extent to the liquid calcium and magnesium I took before arriving at the hospital. I'm sure the month of preparation using Lamaze techniques also helped to contribute to ease the difficult delivery. It is so much better to practice relaxation techniques rather than take pain medicine that is sure to affect the baby. However, if one needs pain medicine during the labor and delivery, they will need a much smaller amount to achieve the desired effect.

After the delivery, Bruce and I rejoiced together at the gift of our new bundle of joy. Neither of us were aware of the challenges which lay ahead.

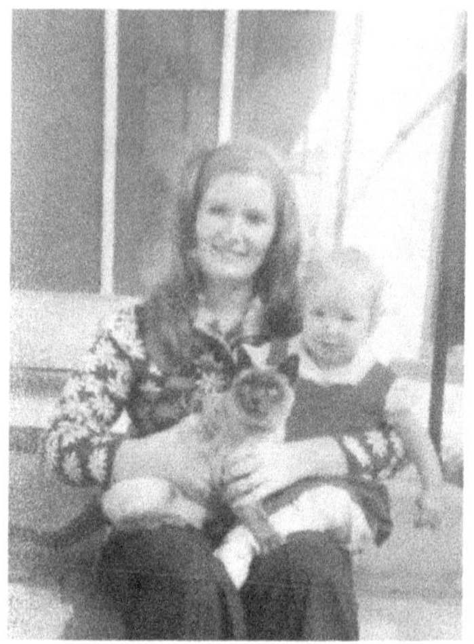

4
____

THE JOYS AND CHALLENGES OF PARENTHOOD

Baby Deborah and I had to stay in the hospital two extra days. Deborah was jaundiced, and had a high bilirubin count. To lower the level in her blood, they placed her under a light for a couple of days. Most children fall asleep under the light, but Deborah cried the entire time, a sign of hyperactivity. When they brought her to me to nurse she was exhausted. About the time she fell asleep, they took her back to the light. Soon her bilirubin count was normal, and they released us.

The proud parents brought the bundle of joy home. She slept for several days, exhausted from the hospital ordeal. My mother-in-law stayed with us for a week and was an enormous help to me. Deborah had Attention Deficit Disorder. She was difficult to handle from infancy. As a first time mother, I felt responsible when she didn't respond to my love and cuddling. The more I tried to soothe her, the harder she cried. Later, I learned that infants with Attention Deficit Disorder could not tolerate that much stimulation; it increased her distress. I felt I failed as a mother.

As the weeks went by it became apparent that our beautiful baby girl became distressed easily. Many times she became more upset when I nursed her. Restaurants asked us to leave several times because we could not calm her down.

When Deborah was three months old I noticed the smell of fresh paint adversely affected her. We were in a rather small library, where they painted the day before. She cried hysterically, totally out of control. Shortly after going outside, she calmed down.

When Deborah was five and one-half months old Bruce and I went to dinner alone on our fourth wedding anniversary. This was the first time we had left her with my parents. She cried for two straight hours. My father-in-law dropped by their house and heard the baby crying. He said, "Give her to me." Yet he also had no luck quieting her. After about an hour, we thrilled three grandparents when the anniversary couple returned.

As she neared one year of age her moods fluctuated. Sometimes she was pleasant and others she threw big temper tantrums. Since scolding only increased her agitation, her father and I placed her in her crib until she settled down. One time she threw a fit because I bought her a pair of velvet coveralls with a ruffled blouse. I assumed she didn't like the straps over her shoulders. She threw a tantrum, and I placed her in her crib, telling her when she settled down she could come out. She screamed hysterically for over an hour before calming down.

I did not know what to do with my beautiful, uncontrollable daughter. Fortunately, a neighbor with a hyperactive son started educate me about hyperactivity. Several other parents who raised children with this disorder shared their experiences with me. I learned it was common to give hyperactive children a drug. The drug calms them, but acts as speed to average adults. I was determined to find another solution.

I started attending a support group led by an M. D. mother of a hyperactive son at Kaiser Hospital in the Walnut Creek, about thirty minutes from Pleasanton. I read a newly released Feingold book that discussed how diet, especially artificial colors and flavors, affected hyperactive children. I felt confident that this program of eliminating artificial coloring, flavorings and certain preservatives could help my daughter. As the doctor/mother talked about her son and the way he acted it became clear that these artificial ingredients affected my daughter. I remembered all the parties I left while nursing her. I got very thirsty while nursing and I drank a lot of that famous red punch everyone served. Soon after, my infant daughter started screaming, forcing me to leave. Naturally, I tried to calm her by nursing, but the red food coloring went through my milk making her inconsolable.

At the support group, I learned of a pediatrician and allergist in Livermore, California. He was also the father of a hyperactive son. He was very sympathetic and worked with hyperactive children without giving them drugs. At the first appointment he injected many common allergens under Deborah's skin and found her allergic to dust and mold. When he injected milk she tried to run out of the building. After I ran to get her, the doctor said he had seen children try to climb the brick wall in his office after he injected them with a substance to which they were very allergic. He tested her for artificial coloring and said in all his years in practice he had seen no one as sensitive to food coloring as my daughter.

He prescribed a year of shots with a combination of her chief allergens. He told me this would increase her resistance to those allergens. Her diagnosis was a cerebral allergy, affecting the brain rather than causing a runny nose or a rash like many affected by allergies.

He took part in a research project using certain homeopathic remedies with hyperactive children and I found it amazing how Deborah reacted to one dose. For over a month my daughter seemed like a different child, an angel. I couldn't believe how quickly she reacted to that remedy. It made me a genuine believer in homeopathy.

This support group suggested I give Deborah no red or any other artificial color for three days and then give her some on the fourth. The test showed parents the tremendous effect of artificial coloring and flavoring on their children. When children have these things all the time it masks their symptoms, and the parent doesn't know what is really bothering their child. We gave Deborah red Kool Aid after three days of no coloring. She was on the floor kicking and screaming within five minutes. Our previously sweet child turned into a Jekyll and Hyde. This was proof for my husband. From that day on he never doubted the sensitivity of his daughter to these things.

We gave her several more homeopathic remedies over the next year. We read all labels checking for certain artificial ingredients, such as flavors and colors. I made all our deserts from scratch. We bought our toothpaste at the health food store. Little did I realize at the time that by removing these artificial flavors and colors, known as carcinogens, I was encouraging the lion to sleep.

In her late 30s, Deborah found out she had an arachnoid cyst in the left front side of her brain. This is not something looked for in the 70s. Many people have them and never know it. This is something she was born with and is very painful for babies. This cyst might explain the A.D.D. and the behavior Connie was talking about.

The Doctors told Deborah to leave it alone. She is happy it doesn't need removing or draining, but it pushes her brain back. The cyst is the size of a plum now.

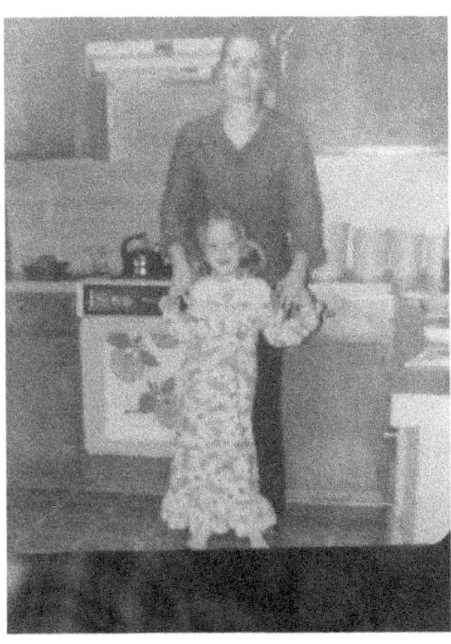

5

ON THE ROAD AGAIN

About a year after the doctor released me from treatment for my first accident, it happened again. I stopped at a red light and the driver behind me drove forward and hit my car, this time a minor incident. However, since I just healed from the first aggravation, it was enough to trigger a relapse. The next day I felt like I had been in a major traffic accident and I required several more months of chiropractic care. Lifting a toddler daily further delayed my healing. Everything seemed fine after the doctor released me. The lion slept for a time.

We relocated to Texas in 1978 when the economy was at its peak and settled in the small town of Splendora, about forty miles north of Houston. We built our first home in a beautiful wooded area. Things were good. Our daughter was doing well with her diet and allergy treatments. We decided in 1980 to have a second child, hoping for a boy.

My lower back hurt during the second trimester of my pregnancy and the pain ran down my right leg. I went to a chiropractor who used a special soft tissue technique, incorporating acupressure. He took no x-rays and used non-force techniques. It relieved my pain, but I needed treatments about three times a week to keep pain free. I ate a healthy diet and took the supplements Adelle Davis recommended in her book *LET'S HAVE HEALTHY CHILDREN.*

Since I expected a rapid delivery, living in the country, over an hour from the hospital concerned us. Therefore, we decided to use a local midwife for a home birth. My doctor agreed to continue seeing me during the pregnancy and made arrangements with the hospital in case complications arose during my pregnancy or delivery. Except for the pain in my right leg, I was in good health.

My mother-in-law flew in from California before the delivery. The exciting day finally arrived, April 3, 1981, after two weeks of false labor. My water broke, and I woke my husband. The midwife arrived in five minutes with oxygen. My husband set up a tripod for a movie camera because we agreed to film the birth for the midwives childbirth classes. I took four tablespoons of my liquid calcium and magnesium and enjoyed homemade chocolate chip cookies my mother-in-law made for the occasion. I delivered a healthy boy who weighed ten pounds, twenty-three inches, one hour after my water broke.

The home birth was a wonderful experience. The midwife came for several false labors. My son did not cry when he was born. He was alert and breathing fine. The birth was a calm and peaceful experience. They wrapped Robert Benjamin MacKenzie quickly in a warm blanket and put him on my stomach to nurse. This is especially important in a home birth since the sucking stimulates the release of a powerful hormone that causes the uterus to contract. What a contrast to my daughter's birth at the hospital. They snatched Deborah away at the hospital for several hours before I even held her. They placed her on a cold metal table with bright lights to clean her up. She cried so hard my husband went over to comfort her. In contrast, his father, grandmother and aunt soon held my son.

Many of our hospitals have made great strides in the development of birthing rooms, with a home bedroom type of environment rather than the sterile and impersonal feeling of regular maternity wards. Birthing centers have become popular. They locate these centers close to a hospital and a state-certified midwife or RN midwife usually runs them. They achieve a homelike atmosphere with the safety of a hospital in close proximity.

In 1975 the United States had only five such centers and in 1996 there were over two hundred of them, showing their growing popularity. Some women still prefer a midwife and a home birth. However, home births are usually not recommended for first births since they are often more difficult.

Regardless of where the new child is born, I believe that a poem I wrote sums up most our feelings at that special time.

LIFE BEGINS

When I see life start anew
It is all that I can do.
To see a brand new face
Oh, what happiness to us it graces.
To hear a faint little cry turn into one great
Big wall
When the new little one makes his presence
Known
To all those to whom he's shown.
With his smiles and his grins
He, your heart will win.
Great big eyes follow you in place
How can you but fall in love with this little face.
From that moment on, we will be glad,
Oh yes, my little one for life with you will
Never be sad.

The lion slept for many years. There was only an occasional movement in its sleep, making its presence known, and then nodding off soundly to sleep again—at least for a little while.

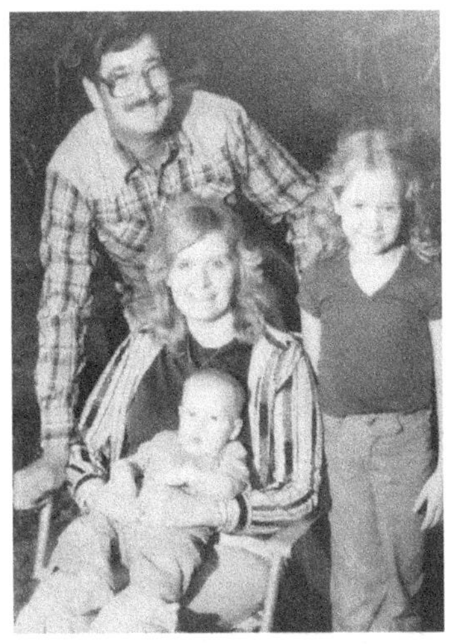

Bruce and Connie MacKenzie, Benjamin MacKenzie and Deborah Benefield

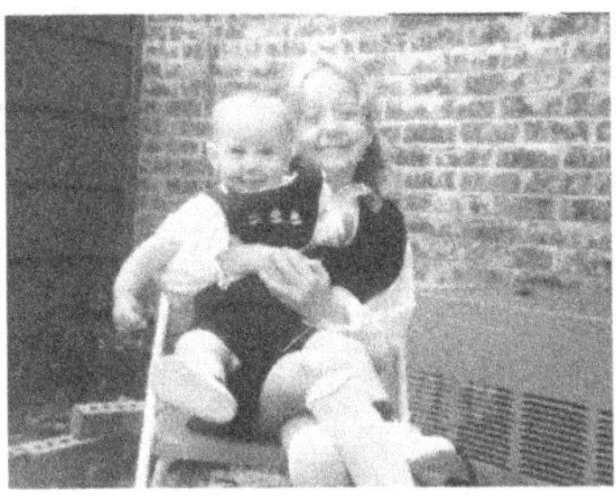

Deborah Benefield and Benjamin MacKenzie

6

THE LION STIRS

I was thirty-five pounds overweight when my son was born in 1981. I joined friends in the improved Weight Watchers program. I reached my goal weight by faithfully attending the weekly lectures and using their eating program. We both received the necessary nutrients, even though I was nursing my son.

After maintaining my weight for several months, I took the training and became a lecturer for Weight Watchers. Over the next three years, I worked with hundreds of people. It was rewarding to help people reach their goal weights. Controlling our weight involves more than counting calories. Many start their new year with a resolution to lose weight. When someone has only a few pounds to lose they reach their goal quickly. However, when someone has twenty-five or even eighty-five pounds to lose, this is not a quick weight loss program. They designed it to change eating habits and behavior patterns.

As their weight decreases and their self-esteem soars, people are transformed. My students learned about themselves and how to cope regardless of their size and shape.

They became more aware of when they use food for comfort or what they hid behind all that weight.

I encouraged my classes to walk and decided to set a good example. I bought comfortable shoes and jogged a mile each morning with a neighbor. My feet pounding on the pavement stirred the lion. I noticed a swelling in my right thigh about a month after taking up jogging. Fear filled my heart, and I prayed it wasn't a tumor.

The mass felt hard and was pliable like a muscle. I told my class I was developing muscles in areas I hadn't noticed before since taking up jogging. I considered why the other leg was not developing the same muscle. I was in denial.

As I prepared my behavior modification lectures, I learned many things that helped me fight off the roaring lion. The five years I spent following a balanced nutritional program of low fat, low sugar, reasonable amounts of starch, three fruits a day and a lot of vegetables helped to prolong the sleep of the lion.

It's interesting to note that a new brochure, *Road Map To Cancer Prevention*, released by M. D. Anderson tells us, "What we eat is related to more cases of cancer than even the cigarettes we smoke. Up to 70 percent of cancers are linked to foods. The good news is that some foods can actually help protect against certain cancers. A low-fat, plant-based diet (fruits, vegetables, grains, and beans) is your best insurance against almost all cancers as well as heart disease."

It goes on to say "People who eat the most fruits and vegetables have only about half the cancer risk for all the major cancers—breast, lung, colon, prostate and cervical—than those who eat the fewest."

Many years before this information became common knowledge there was a wonderful book by George E.

Berkley, Ph.D., 1978, *Cancer—How To Prevent It & How To Help Your doctor Fight It* that shares many little-known research facts that identified nutrition as a powerful tool against the lion. It is exciting that science is researching and finding out why what we eat has such a powerful effect on our immune system's ability to wage war against many of our unseen invaders. The old saying "You are what you eat" takes on new meaning all the time.

Every day a person should eat five to nine servings of fruits and vegetables, six to eleven servings of whole-grain products and two to three servings of low-fat or non-fat dairy products for calcium. Eat a low-fat diet. I followed this basic nutritional program all of those years. Amazingly, what was once far out in left field has been scientifically proven to keep the lion sleeping.

In 1985 my children and I took a two-week vacation to visit my parents in California. My leg was noticeably swollen when I deplaned because the air travel caused swelling of the lymph tissues. It was almost the size of a football. I went to see my old family doctor. Fearing I had a tumor, he wanted to put me in the hospital. I preferred to wait until I got home. He gave me a shot of cortisone, which allowed me to enjoy my visit with a minimum of discomfort.

When I got back home to Houston, the chiropractor took an x-ray of my leg. Fear engulfed me as I viewed the picture. My bone mass was an enormous size, measuring twelve inches, by three inches, by five inches. My upper thigh was more bone than leg. The raging lion consumed most my right thigh.

In 1985, during the economic crash in the "oil rush town of Houston," my husband's business slowed. I had started a plant business, Connie's Touch of Nature, before my California trip. I decided to get my business well established before I having surgery. I worked, even though my chiropractor wanted me to get medical attention. I became intensely involved in alternative health care treatments, including homeopathy, vitamins, massage and herbs. I had a lot of energy and needed it to establish my business. It was a rewarding period of my life. As I poured myself into work, the great escape, I thought my family needed to learn to be more independent since I might not always be with them.

Several months passed since the x-ray and I felt fine. I convinced myself I couldn't have cancer. However, I cried when I looked at the mass and felt like a prisoner in my body with no escape.

Still, I felt I would be victorious. Except for my leg, I was the picture of health. A family friend and physician insisted I go to M. D. Anderson Hospital and see what was wrong. My appointment was in November 1986. An older friend, Lavonne, accompanied me. She had thyroid cancer over thirty years ago and remembered the hopelessness of cancer patients then. They viewed cancer as AIDS is today. They often viewed as contagious and isolated them upon diagnosis. Through her eyes, I saw the improvements in cancer care over the last thirty years.

They ran lab test and accepted my chiropractic x-rays. They scheduled a bone conference for that same day. Lavonne and I entered a room with about twenty doctors. They told me I had the largest bone tumor they had ever seen or read about. They said the type of osteosarcoma I had was most common in teenagers and they wanted to know how I controlled the cancer in my body for so many years. I shared my involvement with alternative health care practices and diet.

After two weeks of testing, my husband and I met with doctors to discuss my available treatment options. The cancer lived nowhere else in my body. They suggested surgery and chemotherapy, hoping the latter would shrink the mass. For months I prepared myself to hear that they wanted to amputate my leg, but on that day, they informed me they needed to take the leg and one-half of my pelvis. What a shock. I would be an invalid for the rest of my life. There were no other alternatives given, so I agreed to the surgery on the condition that they use no blood. My personal beliefs prevented me from taking blood. The doctors said doing the surgery without blood would kill me and refused to do it. Since we were at a standstill, they agreed to follow my case and suggested I return in three months. I left on two legs and feeling victorious. Yet, what was I to do? Where could I go for help?

THE JOURNEY'S ROAD

When I returned months later, the tumor was the same size it had been in the original x-ray the chiropractor took. Strangely, I felt relieved. For years people thought it was all in my head and I did not understand why I was in such pain. I remember wishing there was a picture of my pain so everyone could see what I was feeling. Now I had the picture.

When they diagnosed me with cancer, I assumed I had no control over the disease. That our emotions and thoughts couldn't possibly affect the developing cancer. Or could they? I didn't realize my will to get well could produce such an impact on the lion. After weighing the pros and cons, I decided to fight to live. I decided to see my children grown and raised by their birth parents. I decided to live for Bruce, my-husband and lover for fifteen years. I didn't fear death, but firmly believed I would be a coward if I did not fight to live. It takes a brave person to fight these great odds. Little did I know what all that involved.

In his book *You Can Fight For Your Life* Lawrence LeShan says, "Cancer often kills. Yet there seem to be times when getting cancer can become the beginning of living. The search for one's own being, the discovery of the life one needs to live, can be one of the strongest weapons against disease." Another quote from his book is "Cancer is not just one disease. It is a variety of related diseases that affect different parts of the human body in a diverse number of ways."

It was almost in vogue to have cancer at the time of my diagnosis. Jill Ireland wrote a book describing her trials with breast cancer. Gilda Radner also wrote a book and helped cancer victims find hope and courage. Jill quoted Dr. Simonton in her book. "I think you see cancer as a powerful, dangerous, cunning disease, very difficult to get rid of. It is in fact a very weak disease composed of weak, confused, deformed cells. Its power is the rapidity with which it can grow, multiply and mutilate."

Gilda had ovarian cancer, which has a high fatality rate. Many people still feel a void thinking of Gilda and how she made the baby boomer generation laugh for so many years.

Cancer can occur when our immune system ceases to stop fighting the cancer cells and they reproduce at a faster rate than the body fights them off. When we put undue stress upon our body, we leave it with nothing to defend itself against the rapidly dividing cells and the lion awakens.

Deborah remembers going to her grandma's in California with her mom when she was ten years old. Her brother was with them. He was about three or four years old. Deborah was excited to fly and picked the seats in the back of the plane that didn't lay back. During the flight, Connie cried because she was in so much pain, and Deborah worried about her.

Deborah remembers Connie was in so much pain for the next few days until finally she couldn't take it anymore.

At that point her grandmother took her mother to see the doctor. Deborah will remember that day for the rest of her life. Deborah remembers her mother's leg looked like an oversized football. Connie came home after being told that she had bone cancer in her leg. That shocked everyone, but Deborah didn't understand she was in shock or what was happening. You see, Connie complained the entire trip about the seats that Deborah had picked. When her mother received the cancer diagnosis, Deborah thought because she picked the seats that didn't go down in the back of the plane she caused her mother's cancer.

Upon returning to Houston, they told Connie she had three to six months to live. Deborah remembers seeing her strong dad breakdown and cry. She didn't understand why he cried like that. Soon after, Deborah they told her that her mom would soon die. She didn't understand how the plane and the seats she picked could have caused her mom to get bone cancer, but she mad at herself, and kept thinking she made a huge mistake. She was positive she was the cause for her mom's cancer. It is amazing the way a child's mind twists events, information and trauma. Deborah did not understand she carried that guilt until she began writing her book at thirty-eight years old. It was then her story came into the light.

Deborah truly believes that her guilt is the reason she and her mom experienced so much conflict in their relationship.

CALIFORNIA, HERE I COME

As I debated my next steps, my brother-in-law called from San Diego, California. He told me about a friend of his who, for over twenty years, took people to a leading alternative cancer center across the border from San Diego. They provide an herbal tonic and use other alternative therapies. My friend, Lavonne, took this tonic for many years with good results. I decided to try it. I saw a homeopathic doctor for over a year and was happy to learn the center had one which allowed me to continue my use of homeopathy in addition to the tonic.

I flew to San Diego and spent the evening visiting with Leona. She had breast cancer about twenty years before. She shared success stories with me of those without hope who responded well to their herbal treatment. The next morning as we arrived at the health center it surprised me. The center was a beautiful building on a hillside with a lovely view. There were people from all over the world.

One woman about seventy years old visited the center for around seven years. She looked like she had two noses because of the cancer on her face. When they wanted to do surgery that would almost have left her without a face, she came here. As she spoke my hopes grew. Her smiling face and bright, happy eyes were all I saw. Her condition stayed in remission since she started coming to the center. I met many other long time survivors that day, most of whom standard treatments had written them off. All of them showed a happy and determined spirit.

They provided everyone at the center a diet of no pork, tomatoes, white sugar or bleached white flour. They encouraged us to eat a lot of fruits, vegetables, fish and chicken. The program was similar to the one I followed. They put me on the tonic and I saw the homeopath who prescribed several remedies. I stayed in San Diego with my husband's family. My mother flew in and we embarked on an adventure at a wellness retreat in San Diego for two weeks. We learned a wellness program that affected our lives.

While we were at the retreat my mother asked me, "How long did they give you to live?" As a nurse, she knew doctors told a per how long they had left to live. I told her no one had tried to determine that for me. I was sure it was because by all statistics I should have been in the grave long ago. If they had discovered the cancer many years ago, they would have removed my leg immediately. They can save some limbs today when they find the cancer in its early stages. They view amputation as the best means of treatment in other cases.

At M. D. Anderson Hospital and the alternative therapy centers, they considered my case serious. They offered little hope for survival at this advanced stage, but I had hope. Doctors give fewer verdicts today. With all the research happening in regard to the mind-body connection, Norman Cousin' statement in his book *Anatomy Of An Illness* rings even clearer today. "Other and more comprehensive research studies and experiments will be designed. As a result we will learn a great deal more than we know about the role of the positive emotions and of creativity and of the will to live. Before long, medical researchers may discover that the human brain has a natural drive to sustain the life process and to potentiate the entire body in the fight against pain and disease. When that knowledge is developed, the art and practice of medicine will ascend to a new and higher plateau." Norman Cousins spent the last decade of his life working with some of the best researchers in the world at UCLA to prove this statement.

A neighbor gave me Ann Wigmore's book, *Why Suffer? The Answer? Wheat grass God's Manna!*. She wrote about the benefits of drinking freshly squeezed wheatgrass juice. She shared years of experiences where the health of people improved by eating simple raw fruits, vegetables and wheatgrass juice. Wheatgrass juice was new to me and I didn't run out and buy some, even though the reports were impressive.

Back to the California wellness retreat. My mother and I learned about organic gardening and how pesticides were harmful to our health. We learned about the chemicals in our drinking water, and the benefits of massage and even colonics. In addition, we received a two-week education in stress reduction, the benefits of any type of exercise, and the power of positive thinking.

At the wellness retreat they introduced me to the power of relaxation and visualization. They walked us through the steps, explained the astounding medical benefits of this technique. The doctor shared dramatic blood tests results that showed almost immediate improvement in some of his patients. I relaxed and pictured the seven dwarfs with pick axes singing *Whistle While You Work,* my husband and friend supervising the crew as they whittled my tumor away. The relaxation process was similar to the Lamaze method for childbirth preparation.

After two weeks of wheatgrass juice, fresh fruits and vegetables, I saw a chiropractor and natural hygienist to find an eating program that fit my life. They placed me on a vegetarian diet which included a lot of raw vegetables and fruits, lightly steamed vegetables, brown rice and grains. Frozen yogurt was my weekly treat. For the next two years I followed this eating program. The most popular natural hygienists today are Harvey and Marilyn Diamond, who wrote the best-selling book *Fit For Life*.

I went home with my mother for two weeks. We followed my healthy eating program. We learned about food combinations and the digestive process. We reflected on all the knowledge we gained the last month. I set goals for myself to stay productive and increase my will to live. They told me to rest as much as possible and not to put my full weight on my leg. I used this time to study and learn.

I'd left Texas six weeks ago. Eating at a local salad bar, my mother and I met a girl in a wheelchair. She told us about a nurse teaching a course in acupressure. Acupressure dramatically helped her and told us about the benefits this technique can give in serious situations, especially pain control. My mother and I made plans to take the course the next time I came to California. I arrived home, my arms full of books on conquering cancer, and determination to be well. Nothing could have prepared me for the lion's impact on those at home.

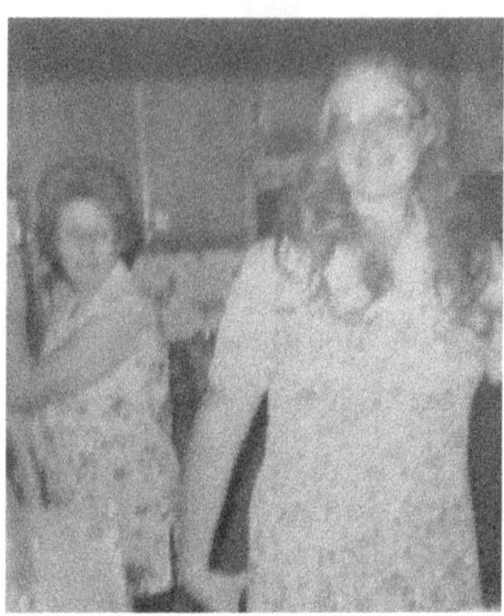

Lucile Dalton and Connie MacKenzie

9

THE HOMECOMING

Imagine returning home to have your eleven-year-old daughter tell you that if something bad would happen to you, it would have been better for it to have happened while you were in California. That was the welcome I received. She said they had already gotten used to me being gone. My mother-in-law told my four-year-old son they had to accept the fact that I was dying and they needed to learn to get on without me.

Soon after my homecoming I went to lunch with a good friend. She said, "What can you say to someone who is going to die?" Three friends came to visit me and apologized for anything they might have done to offend me. They wanted a clean conscience when I died.

I was the living dead; alive but viewed by most of my family and friends as already dead and buried. I wish I could say I was the only lion's victim who experienced this reaction, but it is a common reaction. Lawrence LeShan wrote a lot about this reaction in his book *You Can Fight For Your Life*. "When the family assumes there is no hope and the patient will die, it becomes harder than ever for the patient to have hope and to fight for their life. The family often gives up as a self-protective measure. To some extent it immunizes the family from involvement in the patient's suffering—they are able to tell themselves, 'Well, it will be over soon'." As I read and pondered over these things, I didn't feel so all alone, yet the pain in my heart remained.

For the next two years I followed the program I learned at the center. I also incorporated the knowledge I learned at the wellness retreat. I took my herbal tonic, monthly prescribed homeopathic remedy, freshly squeezed wheat juice each morning and followed my diet plan. I purchased all my fruits and vegetables at a whole foods store to avoid ingesting pesticides and to reap the nutritional benefits of organically grown foods.

In no time at all I went back to California and took the acupressure course. The name of the course was Acu—Pressure connection, implying the involvement of nutrition, exercise and a complete approach to better health. The course is now registered with the state of California. The alternative health care field, also known as complementary medicine, has come a long way.

I enjoyed being with my family, yet I looked forward to the support and encouragement of my mother. Her going through the programs with me made me happy because she joined me in my hope of recovery. We enjoyed the class and practiced with each other. Within two days of starting the acupressure treatments, I noticed a big effect on my leg. A big red patch came up on the tumor mass. I hoped to teach the method to someone in Texas so they could work on me.

After returning to Texas, I became involved in helping others relieve their pain. My pain seemed to diminish as I helped others feel better. I eventually became a certified instructor for the beginning course and started several classes in the Houston area. I also assisted Ival Strom, R. N. the founder, in teaching several advanced classes in Houston.

In 1988 I began massage school. Imagine the teacher's surprise when I told her she needed to teach me from a seated position because I had one of the largest bone tumors in medical history. A friend and I traveled into Houston for training two times a week for the next year. We learned anatomy, physiology, health, hygiene and hydro— therapy. For homework we practiced on several people during the week. We had plenty of volunteers.

I improved, but I still needed to stay off my leg. I continued my appointments at M. D. Anderson Hospital. The mass remained stable, and there was no spreading of the disease. Osteosarcoma usually spreads to the lungs, so they x-rayed my lungs every six months. After each appointment, I returned to the alternative cancer center for more herbal tonic and homeopathic prescriptions.

At one of my appointments at M. D. Anderson, they read my blood work and assumed the results were due to chemotherapy. It puzzled them when they discovered I was not taking chemotherapy. They make many chemotherapy treatments from the same substances found in certain herbs. The disadvantage of chemotherapy is the toxic nature of the product. It kills cancer cells, but also kills the good things a body needs and decreases the immune system. The results are very beneficial when it destroys all the cancer cells. But if we diminish the immune system and the cancer returns, it may cause the person to lose the battle with the lion. When I had surgery, they advised no chemotherapy. If they had advised me to undergo chemotherapy, I would have requested to take part in research projects using immunotherapy. There is exciting progress in cancer therapy research. In 1997 they awarded the American Cancer Society $7,000,000 in chemo-prevention grants.

Tragedy struck in October 1987, three months before I returned to California for my second course in acupressure. My mother died suddenly of heart failure a few months before her seventieth birthday. They treated her for congestive heart failure a year before. Always slim and involved in nutrition, she fell over dead sitting in the doctor's waiting room.

My mother was my mainstay during the roaring lion's attack and we learned so much together. I was glad we spent so much time together over the last year. She would not want grief to overtake me, but she would want me to triumph over the lion. I became even more determined to live.

Mother's father also died of heart failure when he was about the same age. If she exercised regularly, she might have lived longer. She bought jogging shoes and her first blue jeans at sixty-nine years of age. She always said she wouldn't be caught dead in jeans. The things we learned together positively affected the last year of her life. She healed from the head down, but her arteriosclerosis was too advanced to cure. Varicose veins prevented her from participating in many exercises and never learned to swim or ride a bike. We have made significant advances in programs of cardiovascular fitness and prevention. Orthodox medicine has proven that many heart conditions can be reversed by exercise and diet over time.

My seventy-year-old father built the house of his dreams on twenty acres in California after mother's death. He met a sixty-five-year-old, never married, retired school teacher at a square dancing class. He was her Prince Charming. They married five years ago. Dad's sister passed away in her sleep.

He was determined it wouldn't happen to him and took an active part in life.

My mother had beautiful auburn hair. My father and I have strawberry colored hair, Need I say more about my temperament. Lorraine, my stepmother, has a much calmer disposition than my highly excitable mother.

I continued to study and learn about natural health and the science of iridology, or iris analysis. I attended weekly classes for a year to learn about the relationship between the iris and the rest of the body. We learned to identify weak points in the fibers and darkened areas in the iris, which could show problems in the corresponding body areas. Iridology does not name diseases. In European countries they view it as a diagnostic tool, one that is used to help determine what additional testing is needed. Iris analysis is important in preventative medicine. It is a means to determine inherent weakness long before clinical symptoms show up, allowing them to develop a prevention program for the individual.

You can tell how strong your inherited body is by the closeness of the fibers in your iris. We can compare it to fine linen cloth, the closer the weave, the more threads, the stronger the cloth. When a person with a weaker structured body takes better care of himself than stronger structured person he can live as long or longer than the stronger structured one. My iris was closely knit. On a scale of one to ten, I was nine. I'm sure the inherent strength of my body contributed to my surviving such a serious illness.

10

WHEN WE ENDURE TRIALS, WE GROW
BY MILES

They admitted my son to the hospital with bronchitis when he was eight months old. He sounded like a barking dog and could hardly breathe. They allowed me to stay with him in an enclosed room in intensive care since I was still nursing. They moved him to a regular room after twenty-four hours. They thought he might have asthma since it developed during a cold front. Some people call it croup. They told me to be cautious of exposing him to damp air, especially evening air, as he got older. We needed to wait and see what would develop.

A girl friend studied homeopathy for years and read countless books on the subject. She told me about some remedies people found effective. The following year I studied homeopathy, because my daughter's improvement to the remedies her doctor in California prescribed impressed me. There are homeopathic study groups for people to learn to use remedies in acute situations (cold, flu, fever, teething of infants, colic, etc.) all over the United States today. However, in 1982 there was no one in the

Houston area. A close friend shared, she took part in doctor conducted study groups for years in Michigan. It thrilled me. We both lived in Splendora, Texas and formed a study group. We met twice a week for several years to study and research the right remedies for our families.

When the first winter after my son's first attack came, I was well armed with remedies known to help with his previous problems. At the first sign of a problem I rotated three remedies depending on the time of day and his symptoms. The results were wonderful. He is sixteen now and still has to take some of those same remedies if he goes out in the evening air when it is cold and damp. He is usually fine by the next day. Our study group now totaled four. We marveled at how our children's runny noses cleared up and the headaches or cramps of an adolescent girl improved quickly with the correct remedy. Today you can purchase homeopathic remedies in almost any drug store or large chain.

Bacteria are resistant to antibiotics because of the overuse. Old alternative health practices, outmoded with miracle drugs, are taking their place in our healthcare system now. They work by increasing our immune system to fend off foreign invaders. By decreasing our external environmental exposure to pollution, smoke, overuse of prescription drugs, artificial food additives and pesticides we help to keep the lion sleeping. We have made great strides in educating the public about the effects these things have on our immune system's response.

A few years ago the media reported that our children are at risk to harm, when eating large quantities of apples and other fruits prayed with pesticides. Many large chain grocery stores responded by selling organic vegetables and fruits. Many local supermarkets carry organically grown vegetables and fruits today. The public should support their efforts by buying that produce. Yes, we have come a long way in understanding the relationship of our diet to cancer and heart disease.

In 1987 I attended a seminar on natural health in San Diego. The host, Bernard Jensen D.C.N.D. , lectured on nutrition. He shared an experience from the early fifties. He told a group of several hundred people that if they ate more salads, fruits and vegetables they would become healthier. The audience laughed at him and thought it ridiculous that what we eat could have any real impact on our health, especially diseases like cancer. How far we have come.

Many books written by Deepak Chopra, M. D. educate us about the benefits of Ayurveda, an ancient Indian medicine, and how it can help with our modern diseases. Research is being performed in the areas of homeopathy, acupuncture, herbs, massage and nutrition. New books on alternative health care are quite the trend with such books as *Spontaneous Healing,* written by Andrew Weil M. D. helping pave the way for Americans to learn more about complementary medicine.

As the name implies, alternative health care is used to complement our standard orthodox medical care. My children think I'm old-fashioned, and perhaps I am often behind the times. I was investigating the best way to keep the lion at rest. Now, it seems I have unknowingly involved myself in a giant revolution. I'm sure this revolution will end without a definite winner, but a blending of the best of both worlds, orthodox medical care and the age old preventative measures of alternative health care.

11

A NEW CAREER

My husband took over my plant business, and I rested and studied for over two years. I received my Texas massage therapy license in June 1989. My leg remained the same all these years and my health improved dramatically with the alternative health care measures I took. Alternative health care teaches Herrings Law—the body heals from the head down and from the inside out.

In 1989 I was doing so well I started my business. I hired three massage therapists. We worked in a pain and stress clinic with a chiropractor and a physical therapist. It was exciting to see patients responding to the combination of alternative health care techniques such as acupressure, Swedish massage, cranial-sacral therapy and stress diffusion. I formed my own corporation, MacKenzie Medical Rehabilitation Clinics U.S.A. My DBA Total Health and Wellness Clinics were located in Kingwood and Huffman, Texas. It thrilled me to see all the things I learned used under one roof and the wonderful results the patients experienced. Just when all was going so well, the lion raised its ugly head and roared loudly.

It rained, and I still used crutches to keep the weight off of my leg. As I walked to my clinic, my crutches slipped, and I fell backwards. Fortunately, friends caught me so I didn't fall hard on the ground. They helped me inside and massaged me. An ambulance took me to M. D. Anderson. I sprained my back and could not move without excruciating pain.

12

TRIALS AND TRIBULATIONS

I spend the next two weeks in the hospital. The pain immobilized me. While in the hospital, day or night, patients could watch a comedy program on the television. I turned to that station often and thought of how Norman Cousins in *Anatomy of an Illness*, educates that laughter is of significant benefit to help promote the healing process. How true is the old saying that " laughter is the best medicine."

I used the time to read and reflect. In the Carl and Stephanie Simonton and James L. Creighton book, *Getting Well Again*, they wrote " We believe that emotional and mental states play a significant role both in susceptibility to disease, including cancer, and in recovery from all diseases. We believe that cancer is often and indication of problems elsewhere in an individual's life, problems aggravated or compounded by a series of stresses eighteen months prior to the onset of cancer. The cancer patients have typically responded to these problems and stresses with a deep sense of hopelessness, or giving up. This emotional response, we believe, in turn triggers a set of physiological responses that suppress the body's natural defenses and make it suscep-tible to producing abnormal cells."

I asked others recently diagnosed with cancer what unusual stress was in their life six to eighteen months before their diagnosis. They always answered quickly, knowing exactly what their stresses were. I am a believer in the above quote.

Another quote from Carl and Stephanie Simonton and James L. Creighton book, *Getting Well Again*, "... the patient's illness was "psychosomatic". It was 'all in his head', a figment of his 'imagination', and therefore not 'real'. But this is a distortion of the meaning of the word psychosomatic, which simply means that an illness originated as a result of, or is aggravated by, an individual's psychological processes. It does not mean that the illness is any less real because it is not solely physical in origin, if any illness ever is. An ulcer may have originated as a result of, and be aggravated by, anxiety, and tension. This does not make the ulcer any less real."

In their book they explain how as early as 1959 Dr. Eugene P. Pendergrass, president of the American Cancer Society, emphasized the necessity of treating the whole patient, not just the physical manifestations of cancer. Dr. Pendergrass's view underscores the role that psychological factors play in aggravating a disease. It also emphasizes the possibility that psychological factors, including the patient's beliefs, may be mobilized to move toward health. As thoughts and emotions can aggravate physical conditions, they can also contribute to health. Just as someone can become psychosomatically ill, they can move in the oppo-site direction and become psychosomatically healthy.

They continue to relate, based on current medical theory, abnormal cells are occasionally present in everyone's body throughout life. Whether external factors create abnormal cells or they occur naturally, the crucial questions become: What lapse in the body's defenses allows these cells to reproduce into a life-threatening tumor at this time? What inhibits the body's immune system from performing the function that it has performed successfully for years? The Simontons and Creighton give one answer to these questions. "The answers to these questions bring us back to emotional and mental factors in health and illness. The same factors that may determine why one patient lives and another with the identical diagnosis and treatment dies also influence why one person contacts a disease and another does not." I enjoyed reviewing the materials and gained renewed strength to conquer my fear as the lion gained its seemingly powerful hold on my body.

Bernie S. Siegel, M. D. had just released his new book, *Peace, Love & Healing.* I read and reread it during this hospital time. Many doctors noticed the book on their rounds and questioned me about it. Since that time in 1990, M. D. Anderson has had several cancer Survivor Annual Conferences with Dr. Bernie Siegel as the special guest speaker. When I go for my checkups now, there are signs pointing the way to stress and relaxation classes at the hospital. Yes, the revolutionary had at last become mainstream.

A quote from Bernie S. Siegel, M. D.'s book, *Peace, Love, & Healing* sums up this famous surgeon's feelings. "Feelings are chemical and can kill or cure. As a doctor I believe it's my responsibility to help my patients use them to cure and heal themselves. While placebos can be useful, because as symbols of hope they activate expectations, my reputation, my training, my belief in my patients and my own hopeful- ness also have symbolic value, which I can use to guide my patients into health. But I don't see that as a crime. I will always use all the tools at my command, because all healing is scientific. If I'm accused of offering false hope, my answer is that there is no false hope- only false no hope-because we don't know the future for an individual."

After two weeks my back healed enough for me to return home. Little did I realize how much I needed to draw upon those encouraging words in the next few months.

13

AND THE ENEMY ATTACKS

My world fell apart after my return home. I could barely walk with the pain in my back. It took another month before I could walk to the living room.

The doctor associated with my clinic quit and set up his own practice. In 1991 they delayed the long awaited funding. Investors wanted to see the impact of the Iraq-Iranian war. The clinic closed as I recuperated. It devastated me, not knowing if I could revive it.

My teenage daughter and ten-year-old son needed my attention. My husband started working in health insurance sales so he could be home as much as possible with his soon to be bedfast wife and his children. The responsibilities of caring for everyone and everything overwhelmed him. The social worker at M. D. Anderson made arrangements for me to get the services of a home health service agency. The agency provided someone to help me with daily activities at home. They also arranged for me to have a hospital bed, and a portable potty for the duration needed.

Later I had respite care, adult babysitting, while bedridden. My caregivers came in two shifts for about six hours each day except Sunday. They helped me with bathing, dressing, etc. My mother-in-law helped me on Sundays, allowing my family to attend our congregation's Bible meetings. This helped them at this troubled time. They phoned me with the Bible meetings, helping me feel less alone. It is very important for the caregivers of the critically ill family member to seek help, giving them time to re-energize and have the strength to continue.

The sick one benefits from new, cheery faces. Often people not personally involved can give the most encouragement, especially when there are unresolved problems surfacing in the family. How happy I was when one of my caregivers told me she was a longtime cancer survivor. She recovered from a mastectomy many years before and was in very good health. Her aunt was also a cancer survivor who had her leg removed at the hip five years before and was doing fine. That she just returned from a trip to Hawaii gave me hope.

I was fortunate to have a homeopathic doctor as a close friend. She used to come to my clinic to see patients. She called me daily, offered encouragement and suggested remedies to try. She talked to my husband, recommended that he plead with my doctor at M. D. Anderson to consider doing the surgery without blood.

The doctors at M. D. Anderson followed my case over five years. My situation remained stable for four years. They knew the alternative health practices I used and suggested to a Dallas news station that they talk with me regarding the alternative health care approach to cancer. The new station interviewed me in my bedroom shortly after I returned home. I explained how everything stimulated my immune system to fight the cancer and hold it at bay. The fall and the stress of closing my clinic woke the lion!

My homeopathic doctor friend was positive with me during my confinement. She shared stories of patients she witnessed who responded to homeopathic treatment, but still needed surgery to rid themselves completely of cancer. She witnessed many of my alternative practices. A patient introduced her to a homeopathic doctor, and she was so impressed with the patient's results that she learned about homeopathy. If she was right, my body could not destroy the cancer, so it walled it off from the rest of my body to keep it from spreading. My friend knew of the positive results of using your creative energy to help your body fight off serious diseases. For several months she urged me to use my creative energy. My husband bought me a sing along box and I sang. I took up crocheting and made something for everyone I knew. I continued reading, but of a more relaxing nature than the deep study I embarked on for so long. I wrote poetry, and I published three poems.

My husband called the doctor at M. D. Anderson who had been following my case for these last five years. She said she would try to find a doctor to perform my surgery without blood. Fortunately, she was well acquainted with Marvin M. Romsdahl, M.D. Ph.D. and Professor of Surgery for many years. He agreed to meet with me and consider taking my case upon the approval of a conference of physicians. They decided that if my blood raised to normal range they could hyper-dilute it with water and use the cell saver. This new machine circulates the lost blood and returns it back into the body, similar to a kidney dialysis machine.

I believe that when blood is drawn from the body and exposed to the air it should be disposed of, not used for transfusion or any other use. I agreed to their terms since my they were recirculating my blood and not exposing it to the air. It was exactly the same surgery they wanted to do five years before. However, since my diagnosis, the medical world performed a significant amount of research regarding bloodless surgery because of AIDS. I might have died, had tried to perform this surgery years earlier.

Those five years since my diagnosis were productive and rewarding until the last few months. I regretted nothing about my prior decision, yet now I could barely stand because of that mass. My leg became my enemy, I knew it was time to let the leg go. The lion had completely claimed it and it drew strength from my body daily. It was time to say goodbye.

People wonder if they found cancer earlier if they could have saved my leg. The answer is no because of the position of the tumor. If they discovered when I was in my twenties, they would have amputated my leg at the hip. I'm glad kept my leg as long as I did. With early detection, they can avoid many amputations today, but that was not the case so many years ago.

They put me on a new drug, erythropoietin, used to stimulate red blood cell production. It was to help get my blood count up to 12, the level they wanted it before they would perform the surgery. The drug normally works quickly to raise the blood count. My tumor was solid bone and had created an additional feeding source for the mass. It was like having two major arteries going into the leg. The doctors decided they needed to detach the leg and half of the pelvis first. They would cut the artery at the end of the surgery. When they cut the artery, massive amounts of recalculated blood would pour back into me. Hyper-diluting me with water before surgery allowed even more blood to circulate to compensate for any loss. They planned the surgery well and everything depended on raising my blood count from 8 to 12. With the drug, we expected this to occur rapidly.

With renewed hope, I took the erythropoietin, B-12 shots, and iron supplements which also help raise the blood count. By the time my blood count was ready for surgery I was immobile because of the weight of the leg, requiring help just to sit up in bed.

The drug fed the tumor as it increased the red blood cell production. Each day as I lay in bed I could see it grow and the leg became heavier and heavier. Soon I needed someone to help me lift my leg to change positions. My caretaker who had breast cancer years ago gave me homemade blackberry wine, telling me it helped raise her blood count before surgery. I responded to the drugs and the good wine. The wine was the best part. It took two months and three increases in the erythropoietin before my blood count rose to the magic mark of 12.

They scheduled surgery for January 30, 1992. They admitted me several days early for tests and preparation for the surgery. Some friends gave me a wonderful lingerie shower before my admittance. Knowing that they believed I would survive helped give me hope and the strength to go on.

My daughter, now seventeen, had not fared well during my lengthy illness. She felt robbed of her mother during her teenage years and responded with anger. She coped by being an overachiever and threw herself into school and work. She stayed away from home to avoid dealing with my illness. She acted as if I pretended to be sick to receive special attention. She visited me just before they wheeled me off for surgery and broke down crying. She told me she was afraid I would die, sobbing all the while. I told her I absolutely would not die. I hadn't come this far to die now. Later she acknowledged that moment was when she admitted to herself the seriousness of my situation.

At ten years old Deborah shut down. All those years she held her pain inside. She was embarrassed and couldn't handle being at home or around her mother. Deborah truly believes her behavior stemmed from her anger and fear that she caused her mother's cancer.

At college, the day before Connie's surgery, Deborah went in the bathroom at lunch and broke down for the first time. She cried and cried. It was the first time she acknowledged her mother could die. Until then, she fell into her own little world to cope. In her mind, her mom already died. She considered Connie a family member like an aunt or cousin that was living with them.

Growing up with a family member who has cancer affects everyone in the family differently. Someone looking in from the outside, and even others inside with them, can't predict or understand how a person will respond. Each person's experience is unique.

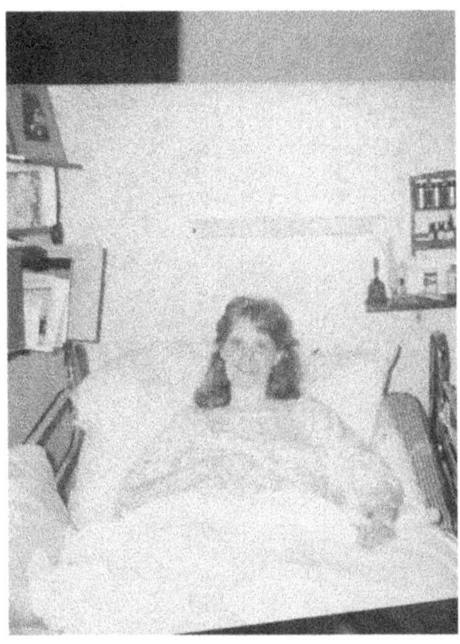

Connie MacKenzie

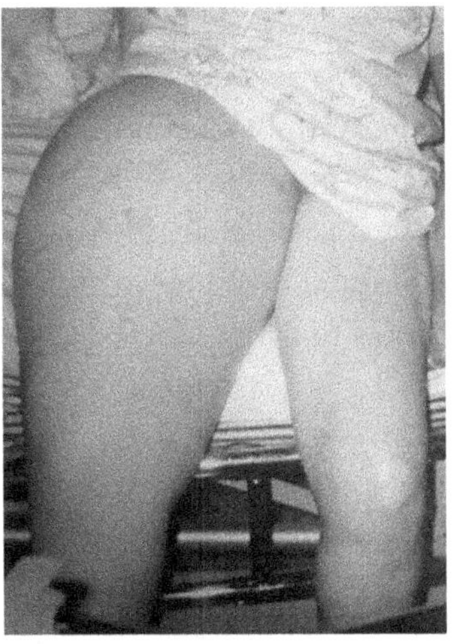

Connie MacKenzie's leg before surgery

14

HOME SWEET HOME

My homecoming was happier than when I returned from California after my diagnosis of cancer. Everyone seemed relieved that the surgery was behind us. My family looked forward to returning to normal, if anyone remembered what normal was like after over ten years of waging war with the lion. My family's positive attitude made me happy. We believed the lion would not return to haunt us. I felt a sense of relief that the battle was over, but I was in for another surprise.

Physical therapy began the week after I came home. With tremendous effort I got to the bathroom without assistance. I wondered how long it would take for me to navigate from one room in my house to another without the wheelchair. The therapist's job was to help me learn how to get up and down from the floor and to use my crutches with one leg. We progressed over the next three months.

My next goal was to acquire my prosthesis. My doctor insisted I master all the skills my therapist gave me before he would prescribe the leg. Remember, I was still rebuilding my strength from being on bedfast for almost a year before my surgery. My progression wasn't as rapid as a normal, active person before surgery. This amputation is one of the most severe of all. Very few therapists had experience with this amputation. My physical therapist and I learned together. Three months passed quickly, and I received the prescription for my artificial leg.

They discouraged patients with this type of surgery from trying to wear a prosthesis. Most were told that they could never wear one. We have made significant improvements in many prosthetic devices during the past fifteen years with lighter metals and improvements in leg parts. Hemipelvectomy patients make up one percent of all amputees, so less research and development has occurred for this type of prosthesis. John Sabolich, in Oklahoma City, has performed outstanding work in developing and improving many prosthetic devices.

Automatic knees are being developed, and a device that provides the wearer with a sense of feeling when the foot touches the ground. It is sad that so many people recovered from this radical surgery are still being told they can't wear a prosthesis. Professionals who make the devices have little experience with this special type and lack the skills necessary to produce a comfortable and usable leg. Fortunately, I lived in the Houston area with one of the largest medical centers in the country. The specialist in prosthetics who made my device had experience working with Hemipelvectomy patients. Yet they only make about four a year. First, they made a plaster of paris mold of my hip area to get the proper fit. When they completed the leg, it weighed twelve pounds with my shoes on. Their goal was to reduce the weight to ten pounds, and they came very close. Before the special, lighter metals, these legs weighed about twenty-two pounds. Imagine lifting and moving that much weight with your rib cage. The rib cage lifts the entire prosthesis since there is no hip or pelvis bone.

My sister, Penny, came from California in May 1992 and we stayed two nights at the Galleria Hotel in Houston. I got everywhere in my wheelchair, and we enjoyed our visit. The outing was a genuine treat.

When I returned home, it was back to the routine physical therapy three times a week and learning to walk with the new leg. The new leg looked beautiful. They designed it to match my good leg. My dad said it looked better than my real leg, quite a compliment for the craftsman. It looked so real, my helper named it Tillie.

To put the prosthesis on, I placed my body into a "bucket" and strapped it around my waist. The bucket has a lightweight leg attached with a hip, thigh, knee, lower leg, ankle, and foot. It took three months to learn to get down on the floor and up again with the leg on. My goal was to walk with a cane, which I accomplished. Learning to walk with the leg was like learning to walk on one stilt. I stubbed the toe to bend the knee. It takes effort to lift the twelve pound leg using the bones under my rib cage. The balance the leg provides me for walking makes it worth the effort.

The force involved with moving my leg made it hard to keep my balance. I resorted to using the three wheeled walker. It amazed me that people have entirely different reactions to my equipment. The three wheel walker reminds people of a scooter and they like it. They also like the electric cart. However, the regular walker and the wheelchair turn many people off since they associate these with a handicapped person.

Many people think the way we feel about ourselves results from how others perceive us. I know the equipment less commonly associated with being handicapped makes people perceive me as less handicapped, which allows them to feel more comfortable. It is like an overweight person is treated in a different manner than someone thinner. Humans are affected by what they see, and it affects how they treat others.

This lesson rang true as I ventured out more, expecting to be treated the same as before my surgery or even before my diagnosis of cancer. I learned that many amputees become recluses and do not fight to be accepted as a whole human being. Many marriages break apart after one mate becomes an amputee. It is hard to realize love can be so shallow, yet the mate also loses a limb and some just recover from it. One statistical survey showed that over one-half of all amputee marriages break up. That is tragic. The amputee and the mate must go together through the stages of grief, denial, anger and acceptance. I knew my husband accepted the loss of my leg when, one night after we made love, he told me he missed 'his' leg. I held him close, but in that moment I knew he completed the acceptance of his loss and our lives could move forward.

I use a wheelchair to moving around my house quickly and can bend over with ease while in it. When I'm away from home, I'm able to climb stairs and go over any terrain with the help of my three wheel walker, which looks something like a tall tricycle without a seat. I look forward to receiving a new leg. They cost over $20,000 and I'm on a waiting list for funds to help with the cost. It is frustrating that lack of funds for the proper equipment. It keeps me from being a more productive member of our society. Medicaid doesn't even pay for a pair of crutches if you are over eighteen and have a long-standing condition. I'm grateful to Texas Rehabilitation for providing me with my leg, a lift for my car and recently an electric cart so I can get around in my neighborhood, at the mall or a day at the zoo. A United Way Agency paid for my home physical therapist who made my physical rehabilitation possible. I thank the agencies which help many like me to have a life of independence.

One poem I wrote came to my mind.

LIFE IS MINE

I began to know what was mine
When I was in my prime.
To live and be who you are
yet know you still will travel far.
As we live we hope to earn no scorn
for this our life we were born.
When the last page has been turned
let's hope that we have learned.

15

A NEW JOURNEY'S CHALLENGE

Unfortunately, society views amputees differently. I noticed people respond more favorably when I wear my prosthesis. A child adapts more easily to the loss of a limb because they are agile and more athletically inclined. The older the amputee, the harder it is to adjust. With the advances in prosthetic devices those with the use of their knee and upper leg, or even when a portion above the knee has been removed, do better with an artificial leg. Why, they even run. When the hip remains the amputee has more use of the leg than someone with no hip and only half of a pelvis.

Well-intentioned friends compared me with those who had an amputation below the knee and expected my progress to be the same. My improvement disappointed my daughter. Of course, she was unhappy that her mother differed from other people and realized I always would.

I came a long way. I conquered the lion, and the situation I found myself in made fighting the lion seem like child's play. My new goal was to regain acceptance in society as a contributing human, even though I lacked a leg. I knew achieving acceptance would not be a simple task. I wrote several poems when bedfast and my mind referred to these thoughts to help me through this difficult time. I hope you enjoy them.

NEVER LOOK BACK

Never look back to yesterdays sorrow
For life begins anew tomorrow
For today is not a part of yesterdays trials and strife.
Our life is not what was, but what is to be.
So never be afraid to follow your dreams
No matter how impossible it seems.
We are responsible to live each day no matter what it brings.
To mourn and to mope offers us no hope
So give each day your most.
Then see what happiness your life will invoke.

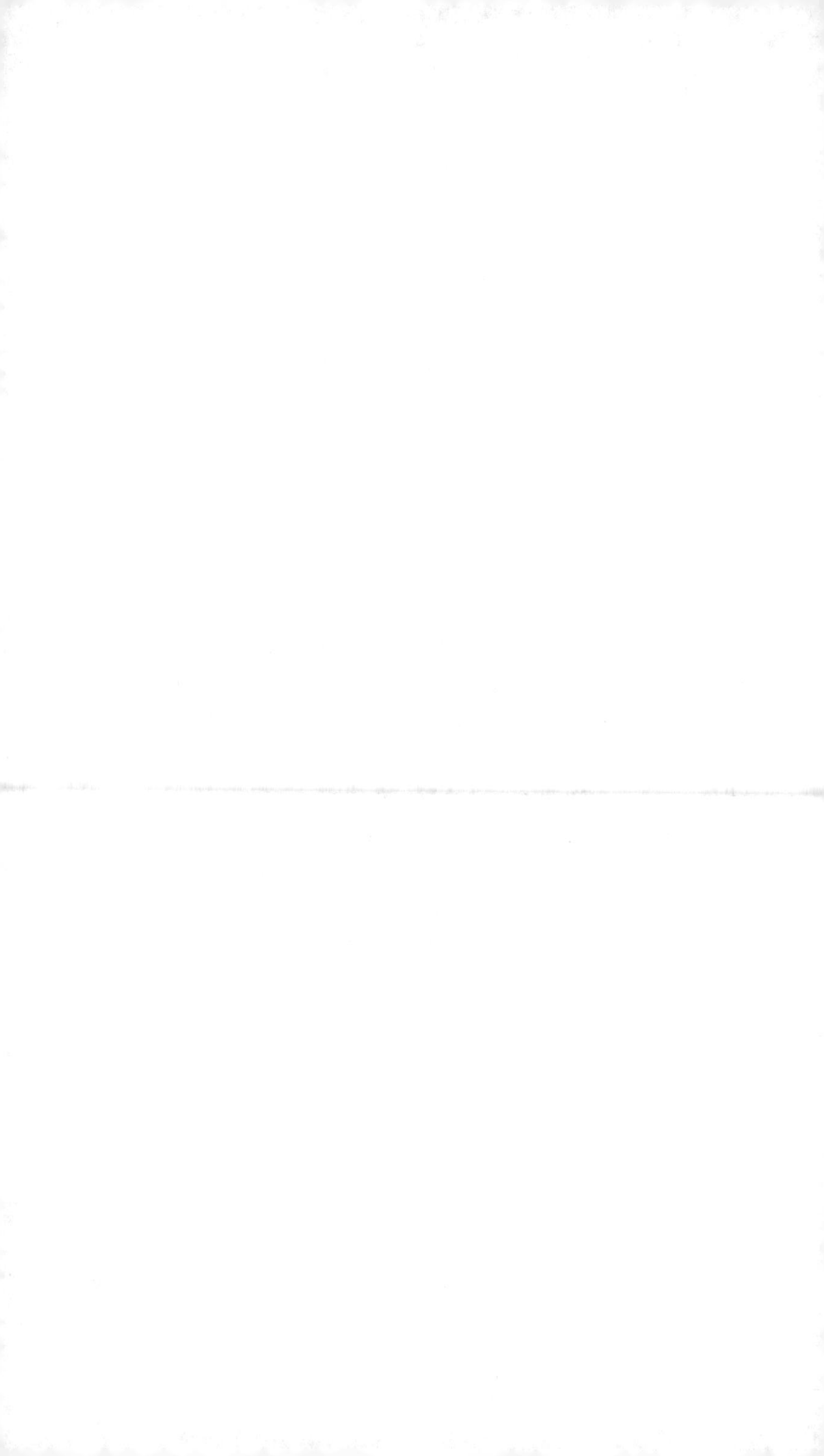

COURAGE WILL GET US THROUGH

Courage, no matter how small
It will help us most of all.
We can make it through tomorrow
If our heart will let us borrow.,
Strength will be renewed so ever let us follow.
To dream to do what's right
Let's not give up the fight.
To end the wrong and sing a song of happiness and light.
So, go on and show courage,
Never become discouraged
For we can start anew in all the things we do.

THE GREATEST GAME OF ALL

When I recall the greatest game of all
It began when I was very small.
Yes, life with all its pain and sorrow
Yet we have much hope for tomorrow.
To live with no problems, we might neglect to reflect
And not become understanding as of yet.
As we go through trials
We will grow by miles.
To pass through a storm and not be overturned
From this our heart will learn.
Then we will yearn for a better day
When we will have our way.
And we can say regardless of the rest that we survived
To thrive in the game of being alive.

I suppose everyone wishes to thrive in the game of life. However, many amputees say other people's attitudes change when they see someone without a limb. I noticed a big improvement in people's attitude toward me once I had my artificial leg and had mastered using it. People who meet me now don't know I'm missing a leg when I wear my prosthesis.

If only people realized what is required of someone with physical challenges to prove their competency. People seemed viewed me with less of a brain because I lost my leg and hip. An African American friend summed it up nicely one evening after laying my feelings open to her. She said she was not physically challenged, however, by being a woman and African American she knew she had to excel at a higher level than her white or male co-workers to receive the same pay or position. A light switched on in my brain. I realized I was now part of an extreme minority and faced the prejudice of others.

In Hitler's reign they quickly disposed of the handicapped. They rounded up the handicapped and didn't give them a chance to prove their worth as human beings. Just imagine if Helen Keller or Mozart lived in Germany during his reign. He would have killed them because of their physical disabilities. We need to learn to look beyond the outside appearance and not place people in a worthless category. We often treat a person in a wheelchair or with an amputation like someone old and frail, ready to be put out to pasture.

What a tragedy the young don't appreciate what people in their seventies, eighties and older offer the younger generations. Though the world differs from their younger years, we still experience the same basic joys and sorrows. And though in some ways things are more difficult in our modern world than they were in theirs, we can still learn a lot from our older role models. The character portrayed by Jessica Tandy in "Fried Green Tomatoes" is an example of this. The whole movie was about a friendship she developed with a much younger, middle-aged woman. What the younger woman learned from the older woman's life experiences taught her to cope with her current problems.

When I reached forty, I rejoiced that I lived that long. After all, they diagnosed me with cancer at thirty-three years of age. How sad that our society worships youth rather than appreciating the wisdom of older people. It is said that knowledge is the collecting of facts, but wisdom is the application of those facts. Yes, it's not what we learn, but how we use it that counts in life. In the works of Shakespeare, "Of all knowledge, the wise and good seek most to know themselves". Marcus Aurelius said, "It is not death that man should fear, but he should fear never beginning to live at all".

I had the privilege of friendship with two people who lived to be one hundred. They both took joy in living. One always bounced back, even after breaking a hip twice and needing several operations over the years. Her mind was clear until the last few months of her life. The other was also clear thinking until her last year. These women made a goal to live to be one hundred years of age and they accomplished it with joy and determination. Let me add they also had a supportive family and good genes.

In his book, Bernie S. Siegel recounts a few years ago gerontologist Ken Dychtwald asked hundreds of people, "How old do you want to be before you die?" The majority didn't want to live past sixty- or sixty-five. They assumed their lives then would be devoid of play, sex, independence, or meaning and filled with problems. The elderly, however, wanted more years. And women generally wanted more years than men.

"The answers all depend on whether or not you feel in control of your life and thus whether you look forward to the future with hope or with fear. One ECaP (Exceptional Cancer Patient) member, a wonderful ninety-two year old woman named Shirley, joined his group. Once, when everyone was talking about how afraid they were of cancer, pain, dying and so on I asked her, 'Shirley, what are you afraid of?' She said, 'Driving on the parkway at night.' That put the other group members' fears to rest because she had lived through everything they are still afraid of except death. Remember, if you decide to live to be one hundred loved ones may die before you. It takes courage to survive and be 'the last apple on the tree', as one of my patients said."

It would be so wonderful if every newly diagnosed person with cancer could be in a support group conducted by Bernie Siegel, M.D. It infuriates me that offering hope and comfort during terminal diseases is in such short supply. We can put a man on the moon, yet we haven't learned how to help give peace to someone dying. Many view assisted suicide as the only solution. Some considered it a favor to help me commit suicide as I lay suffering in bed. How glad I am for the good caretakers and friends who encouraged and comforted me, giving me the strength to go on.

What a contrast to a TV news report given about a woman confined to a wheelchair at age fifty-two. Her husband encouraged her to choose a day to die. According to the interview, her husband wanted her to choose the 4th of July because Independence Day was their anniversary. He said it would be her gift to him. According to her therapist, she had a renewed desire to live and wanted to go out and enjoy life. On the evening before July 4[th,] her caretaker and husband of many years prepared a poison drink and handed it to her. He turned on the movie, "Forrest Gump," and went to bed, leaving her to die alone. The report ended saying his case never came to trial and after four months in jail and he was a free man. He is now a speaker for the Hemlock group encouraging people to help their loved ones commit suicide. How can an evidently devoted husband of so many years turn into an assistant of murder? As I mentioned before, it is important for the caretakers to get relief assistance to allow them to revive their own strength and energy so they don't become worn down by the demands of caring for a very ill person.

Norman Cousins in his book *The Anatomy of An Illness* shared, "Death is not the ultimate tragedy of life. The ultimate tragedy is depersonalization—dying in an alien and sterile area... separated from the spiritual nourishment that comes from being able to reach out to a loving hand, separated from a desire to experience the things that make life worth living, separated from hope." When Norman Cousins wrote this there was no hospice care as we know it today. This movement helped give dignity back to the dying and encouragement to their loved ones.

A quote from *Love, Medicine and Miracles*, "All of us, especially those who are living with serious illness or trauma, are constantly balancing the rewards of life versus the 'cost of living'... Death is not the worst thing. Life without love is far worse." Having mastered the art of living day by day, we can always manage twenty-four hours when we have an important goal to reach.

Dr. Siegel goes on to say, "In a pep talk on this subject to Melanie, a nurse with breast cancer, I said, 'this postponement can last a long time.' She said, ' You don't have to tell me that. My mother came home one day when I was sixteen and said, 'Girls, I've been told I have leukemia and that I'm going to die within a year. But I'm not going to die until you're all married and out of the house.' Eight years later she attended her youngest daughter's wedding." What a fine example of one who kept living despite the odds against her.

16

THE RIGHT TO CHOOSE

Bernie Siegal, M.D talks about the will to live and the choosing of letting go in a peaceful death, yet not one that is an assisted suicide. His grandfather, at ninety-one, told his family to get his friends together because he would die that night. "To humor him, the family complied. That night after the party he went upstairs, lay down, and died."

He shares a word of advice to all of us in this thought: "Each of us had that option. I might choose to live when someone else might choose to die, but that depends on what we need to accomplish and how much loving remains to be done. Death is no longer a failure but a natural option and, since I have redefined myself as a healer and teacher, I can participate in this choice and help patients to keep on living until they die. We must realize people are not living or dying but alive or dead. Label someone terminal and he is treated as dead. This is wrong; if you are alive you can still partici- pate by loving, laughing and living. Before I would accept a quadriplegic's decision to die I would have him take one month of art lessons from another quadriplegic who does incredibly beautiful painting holding the brush in his mouth."

My wish, as a former cancer patient, is for the family of critically ill people to encourage and support the patient's efforts to live. When their will to live is gone, help them by giving support and permission for the loved one to let go, but not by suicide. This way they can go in peace with the love and comfort of their family. We see this today in many hospice situations. They hold severe pain to a minimum in this atmosphere of love.

They have developed many new techniques to keep terminal cancer patients relatively pain free and clear headed during their last days. One way is by putting a pain killer pump directly into the affected area. Many times homeopathic remedies, given in the proper dosages, have been reported to make the patient more comfortable during their final hours. There are several remedies which when given to the family members help them through this time. Yes, much can be done to make a peaceful passing in love possible for our critically ill loved ones without resorting to assisted suicide.

17

SLOWLY, STEP BY STEP

Within one year of my surgery I completed the physical therapy to function with and without a leg. They told me I would continue learning to be more adept at doing certain tasks and eventually I would drive an automobile and be confident going out alone. At the time I had doubts that I could ever do much alone again. Sometimes I needed help just getting my leg on and off to go to the bathroom. Yes, I had to remove it every time I used the restroom. After a while I felt as if I had passed a college course, like mastering the Obstacles of Bathroom 101. Bathrooms come in many shapes and sizes in private homes and public facilities. There are high and low toilets, grab bars and no grab bars, etc. Depending on the layout of the room, I might have something to lean my leg against. When the wall was on the right side I had it made. When it was on the left, I had nothing to lean on to help me balance as I put on my leg. By January 1994, I became an expert and I felt ready to conquer the rest of the world.

Even today, when I'm going somewhere I have never been before, I often need to figure out how to get into a building. They design most to be handicap accessible, but it is unbelievable that some of them have steep ramps the handicapped person can't maneuver when they are alone. Many times the bathroom doors are heavy and open in the wrong direction for the person in the chair to open it. Sometimes I need to ask a stranger for assistance.

I responded to an ad in the newspaper by a doctor looking for people to work with him in a nutritional business. We met, and I signed my name on the dotted line to become a distributor in the multi-level marketing company. I ran ads and gave small nutrition classes at my home with the aid of a video. This helped me regain some confidence in my professional abilities, but I found it difficult to build up the business since I was not driving. Once a month I went into Houston for special training meetings. It was a special treat when the doctor sent me to Boston with his wife, a registered nurse. He had an emergency and couldn't go. He called me to say I had one day to get packed. I was thrilled.

We stayed in Boston four days and I became well acquainted with the Hilton Hotel. Supervised outings, such as this one helped me become more independent and prepared me for going into the big world all alone.

I stayed with the nutritional business for almost two years and benefited in many ways. It cost me to work each year as I never made a profit. My family's financial difficulties unfortunately meant I couldn't afford to stay with the program. It was a sad decision because I received a lot of satisfaction being active in the nutritional field again.

Our daughter became a cosmetologist and esthetician within one year of graduating from high school. Shortly thereafter, she moved away from home. She felt that she was old enough to eat anything she wanted and as a result she felt miserable most of the time. Like many of us when we are young, she knew all her problems would be solved when she was on our own.

A famous news commentator recounted that his father was an amputee before his birth. He reported on his feelings growing up and described how he wished his father could play ball with him and be more like the other kids' fathers. He researched and found that many times children of parents with an amputation are super achievers, evidently trying to make up for some perceived weakness in their parents. When Deborah was twenty-two the department store she worked for became the top producer in the nation for the line of skin care products she managed. She was a very hard worker and excelled despite her A.D.D. She had grown up a lot in the last few years and realized that when she ate foods with coloring or was around strong fragrances for long periods of time, she became nervous and irritable. She reacted with powerful mood swings when she ate things she was sensitive to. I wish children with Attention Deficit Disorder grew out of it, but unfortunately many remain affected throughout life.

Those artificial colorings and flavorings are everywhere. One reason most people don't realize the effect they have on their children because they stay in their system for three days. The odds are a child will ingest more coloring in food during that time and they will notice no change. As a parent, I know it is worth the effort involved to avoid them in the diet's of children's with A.D.D. It is easier to avoid these things today thanks to better food labeling and food manufacturers providing us with more natural flavorings and coloring in their products.

I have been fortunate to have the services of the home health agency. For the last three years Judy has helped me with tasks difficult for me to like making the bed and mopping. She has also been my confidant, cheerleader and friend. She encouraged me when the frustrations of rehabilitation started to get the best of me. As I mentioned previously, many times someone outside the family circle, who doesn't deal with the situation twenty-four hours a day, can give support the family may not be able to provide.

One of my daughter's chief complaints was that I didn't drive anymore. It delighted her when in the summer of 1995 a friend sold me a good used car and I started driving. It terrified my husband for me to be out alone and it took awhile for them to quit worrying about me entire time I was out. One day when I was out alone my car broke down. I got help and had the car taken to the garage for repairs. When I got home, my son said. "Mom, you handled it just like a real person!" Yes, maybe I was on my way to being accepted as a real, whole person again.

The friend who sold me the car wanted me to join her in water aerobics at a health club near our home. We started going to classes in the summer of 1995. I swam a few times since my surgery and the water was such a wonderful equalizer I knew I could participate in the classes. People didn't even know I had one leg when I was in the water. Swimming was always one of my favorite sports and I'm so glad I could still take part. It took me awhile to be comfortable getting around the club, but I soon felt right at home. People approached me and tell me how I inspired them to keep working out. At first I could tell it shocked many to see a legged lady at the gym in her wheelchair and swim suit. Soon they wondered about me if they hadn't seen me in a while. I cannot emphasize enough how much the water exercise helped with my balance and increased my strength.

Initially, someone had to take my wheelchair in and out

of the car for me. I drove to the gym, honked, and someone quickly came out and helped me unload it. It was wonderful when I received a lift for my car. How I surprised everyone when they saw what appeared to be a luggage compartment on top of my car come down with the wheelchair attached. I truly had my independence.

In the spring of 1995 a friend since the third grade sent me tickets to California. I had not been home in over eight years and I went all by myself. Once I arrived in California, I had a lot of help from all of my friends who lived between Modesto and Eureka. It was a lovely trip and helped me become more confident in my ability to go places alone. Each home I stayed in was a fresh challenge. Two of my friends had two-story homes, and we had quite a time carrying the wheelchair up and down the different levels. I learned it was easy to scoot up and down the stairs on my behind. The three weeks flew, and it was time to return home to Texas and my waiting family.

Before my surgery, I had a large clientele as a licensed massage therapist. Now most people failed to see how a physically challenged person could help them get better. There were some treatments I couldn't do because of the severity of my surgery, but I did fine work on my family and a few close friends. I tried, but was unable to build up a practice. I decided to specialize in different areas of the health field, ones that didn't require as much physical effort. I received a scholarship with the British Institute of Homeopathy and am started the course. I also worked on my naturopathy degree from a school in Illinois. I looked forward to using these tools to help others become more educated in preventative health care. It did my heart good to help others learn about the things helped keep the lion sleeping.

They expect to diagnose half of us with cancer in our lives, but we all have cells that could become cancerous each day. It is my sincere desire that with the joint efforts of orthodox and alternative health care professions if we cannot destroy the raging lion, we can be armed with the proper knowledge to keep him sleeping.

Deborah and her dad both knew how her mother's rehabilitation was hard on the entire family, especially the restroom struggles. Connie's husband invented a medical device to help her in the bathroom. Both Connie and her caretaker found the device beneficial. When Deborah saw it she and wanted to help her dad. They have a patent and are still working on getting it on the market.

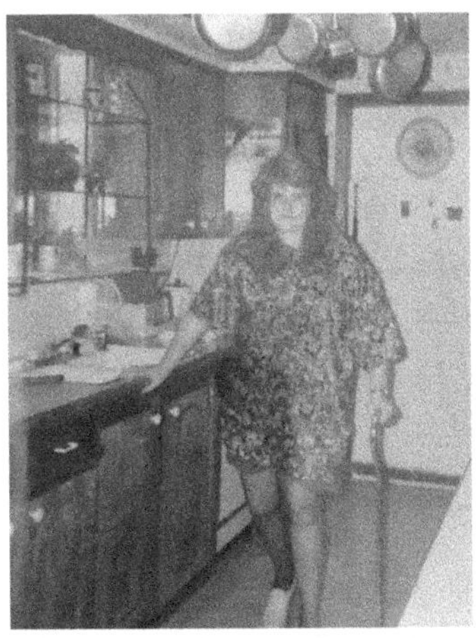

Connie MacKenzie

18

MANY TO THANK

How grateful I am that my doctors at M. D. Anderson followed my case all those many years and offered so much encouragement. I was fortunate to have kind men and women of orthodox and alternative health care professions who some considered in opposing camps. They worked as a team to keep the lion sleeping. Both sides seemed surprised at the many years of my remission. The doctors in Mexico who specialized in alternative health care told me to never turn my back on my orthodox care providers since they never turned their backs on me.

Unfortunately, this happened to many who used alternative health care a few years ago. They often cut people off from orthodox care when they availed themselves of help in non-traditional forms. Fortunately, this is rarely heard of today. Many fine research hospitals are studying the alternative health care disciplines. They are encouraging the use of nutrition, relaxation, visualization, homeopathy, massage, acupuncture and many other fields now considered complementary medicine in the patients' fight against the raging lion, cancer. What a wonderful day it will be when, as in China, orthodox medicine and alternative health care providers work alongside each other to utilize the strengths of each and finally put the lion to rest.

A milestone day occurred in February 1997. It was five years since my surgery and it was time for my checkup. My original diagnosis was ten years prior. You can imagine my joy when my blood work came back with results near perfect and the x-rays of my lungs were clear. I gave Doctor Romsdahl, the brave surgeon who took my case when others would not, an enormous hug of gratitude for the gift of life that he gave back to me. In appreciation, I left him a copy of one of my poems.

THE GIFT OF LIFE

The most wonderful gift of all is one that gives meaning
even to the small.

To be able to bat a ball or play with a doll, small children
rejoice in it all.

Why when we grow tall do we forget how wonderful it is to
be alive at all.

To enjoy seeing the season change one by one even summer,
winter of fall.

To find life's joy even amidst the hustle and bustle of a busy
mall.

See the people short, fat and tall.

Upon their faces you see traces of happiness and sorrow;
watch them all.

If only we can remember to recall, the most precious gift is
life, so let's enjoy it one and all.

As my husband and I left the hospital, we paused in the main lobby to listen to a fine musician playing a beautiful piano. What an uplifting experience for the patients and their families to hear music, which encourages the stimulation of their own immune system to help defend itself against the attack of the lion. Yes, how far we have come and how the gap between orthodox medicine and alternative health care is narrowing.

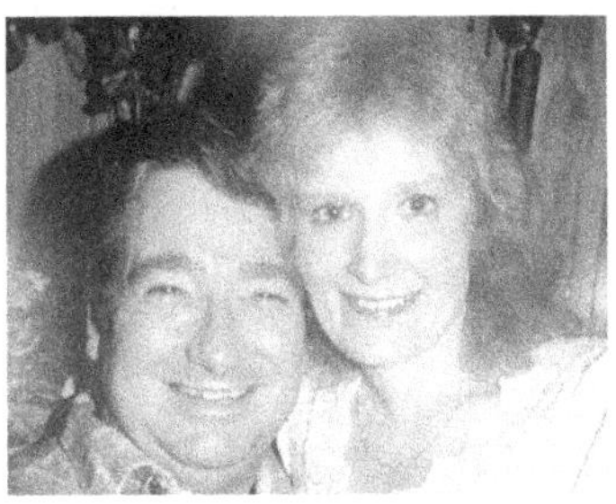

Bruce and Connie MacKenzie

19

WHAT HAPPENS TO CONNIE NEXT?

After they removed her leg and hip, she received great news. The lion vanished. She was thrilled it was over, as was her family. Or so they thought.

Deborah moved to San Francisco, California, for her work. She remembers receiving a call one morning. Her mother's cancer was back. This time the lion roared. The lion took up residence in two places in Connie's brain. Once again, a shock to everyone. The brain, really? How could this be?

Everyone thought the leg and hip was bad; her tumor weighed 69 pounds and looked like two large watermelons connected. Did Connie deserve more? Connie, however, kept doing all her healthy eating and cared for herself. She really had come a long way.

Deborah's mind was blank, and she once again threw herself in work as an escape. She returned for a week to be with her mom during the first brain operation at M.D. Anderson in Houston, Texas. There they removed the front part of Connie's skull, replacing the bone with plastic. The first operation went so well they scheduled the second one two months later.

The second surgery removed the back section of her skull, replacing the bone with plastic. Unlike the first operation, this one was difficult. The changes became apparent quickly. Connie became forgetful, and eventually she reached the point she spoke at the level of an eight-year-old.

Along the journey Connie found out the lion settled in her collarbone, then later her baby finger. For Deborah, the baby finger was the hardest. Connie heard her tears over the phone and said "Why are you crying Deborah, this is no big deal. My baby finger is nothing. It has to be cut off." To this day, Deborah doesn't know why that hit her so hard.

Eventually, Connie included the use of radiation and chemotherapy. However, her family knows it was her will to live, her searching for everything she could get her hands on, and her desire to find alternative way of life that kept her alive.

After the second brain surgery, she went in and out. Deborah's dad (her Prince Charming) took fantastic care of Connie for forty-six years.

We were all in the hospital; in shock. Connie was alert, open, talking, and memory had come back. Two weeks later, at a conference in Florida, Deborah received a call informing her Connie was in hospice. She remembers, in the hospital, her mom telling her she wanted her own bed. Over the phone Deborah said, "I love you mom." Connie said she did too. Deborah flew back to Houston a spent nine more days with mom in hospice care. January 8, 2018, Connie passed in her bed with her family around her; just the way she wanted to go.

Deborah is glad her mom didn't die from cancer. Connie was told at thirty-three she had months to live. She lived to the age of sixty-five. Connie died because of a staph infection and pneumonia that picked up in the nursing home. She had only been in the nursing home one week.

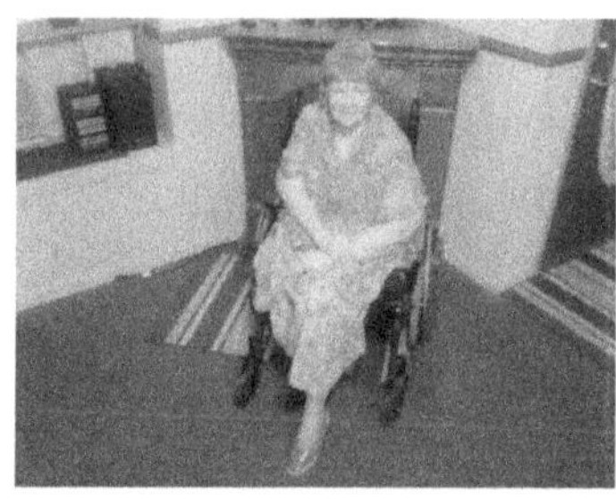

Connie MacKenzie

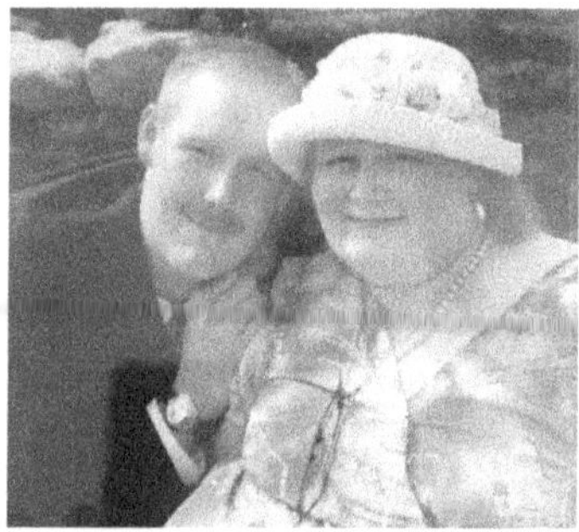

Benjamin MacKenzie and Connie MacKenzie

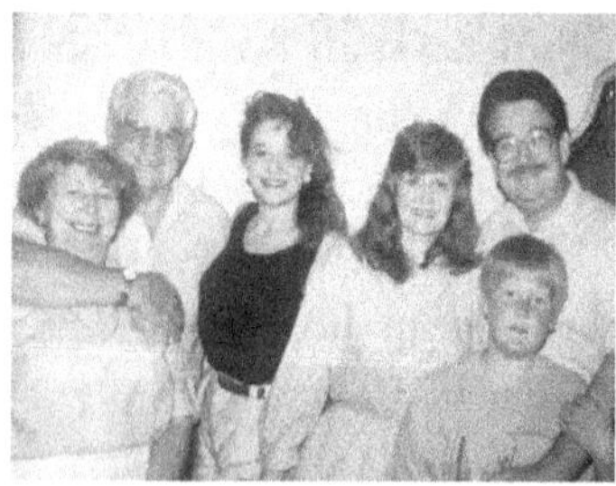

Ben and Lorraine Dalton, Deborah Benefield, Connie, Bruce and Benjamin MacKenzie

20

SOME FINAL THOUGHTS

I am so happy her story is out. It was time. It was her wish, her dream to share this with you and I hope it brings you encouragement. No matter where you are in your cancer journey, please know that no matter how down you get, how much pain you are in, you are still a gift to the world.

My story is ongoing. I am just now beginning to discover all the ways this experience has impacted my actions and my life. I'm sure there is so much more I will learn and eventually share.

If you have family struggling, and they find it difficult to deal with the illness, never take it personally. Know they are trying to be strong for you. They may push you away or focus on work or something else. It has nothing to do with you personally. They may struggle to express how they feel, or they may avoid putting any extra burden on you. They may try to start a fight with you, or those around them. They may say mean things they do not mean. They are in emotional pain. Thinking you may lose a person you love is almost too hard to bear. Pushing you away may be their way of preparing for your death. It may be the only way they can keep it together for you in the present. I blocked my mom out. I started fights. I made her feel horrible. I found ways to stay away and sometimes I wished it was over. Even when I didn't want it over. I wanted the pain and anger to stop and I didn't know how to make that happen. Even when they don't show how much care as often as you hoped, thank them for the support they give and the love they show. Ask them to seek support and help.

Focus on yourself and make yourself better. You can't control or change the behavior of others. Keep your spirits up, find a hobby that makes you happy. Give yourself permission to stay in bed an entire week after going to the doctor or out to lunch with a friend if that is what you need. It's okay. Don't push yourself because you want to make others happy.

You may lose friendships and people you thought would be beside you may not show. They probably don't know how to handle the situation and they don't want you to see them breakdown. Most of all, they don't want to upset you.

If you are in a toxic relationship and are being abused, please get help. You deserve better. There are programs, hotlines and support out there. Remember, you are more important. You are fighting for your life! Keep negative energy away from you and surround yourself with positive people. If you can't find positive people, create that space within yourself. Watch movies and read books that make you feel happy and strong. Seek your own answers, but do it wisely. Never allow your circumstances to make you a victim. You control your thoughts and actions every day, make them positive. What can you do right now, even from your bed, to help others? What can you do to inspire others?

Journal your story. There are people out there who will help you publish it.

When talking with cancer patients about this book, the number one thing I heard was: Just one story that brings hope, one story that shows someone who didn't give up, one story that brings comfort to my day, encourages me to get through the next day.

With much love for you and your family on this journey.

Connie and Deborah

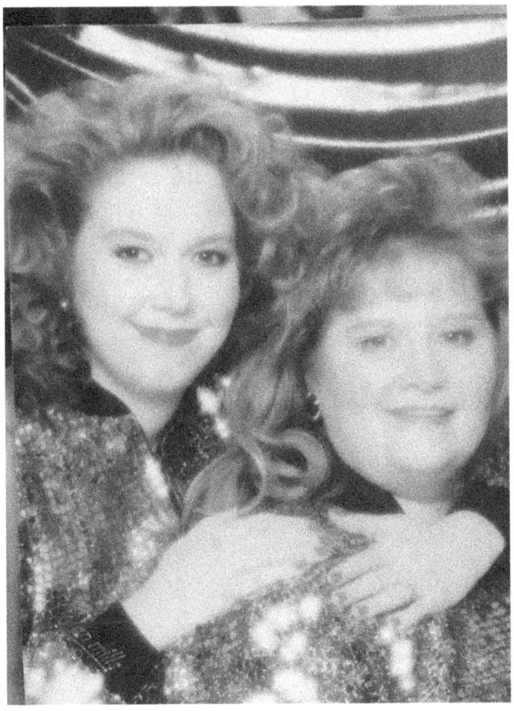

Deborah Benefield and Connie MacKenzie